STRETCHING

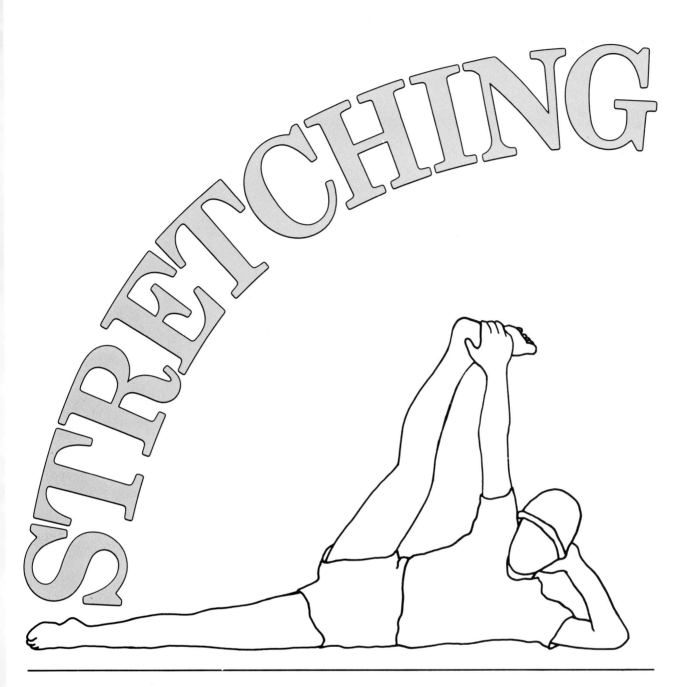

by BOB ANDERSON
Illustrated by JEAN ANDERSON

SHELTER PUBLICATIONS, INC.
BOLINAS, CALIFORNIA, USA

Shelter Publications, Inc..
P.O. Box 279
Bolinas, California 94924 USA

Distributed in the United States by Random
House and in Canada by Random House
of Canada Ltd.

**Library of Congress
Cataloging in Publication Data**

Anderson, Bob, 1945-
    Stretching.

    Includes index.
    1. Exercise. 2. Stretch (Physiology) I. Title.
RA781.A59   1980   613.7'1   79-5567
ISBN 0-936070-01-3
ISBN 0-394-73874-8 (Random House)

First printing, January 1980
Second printing, July 1980
Third printing, September 1980
Fourth printing, December 1980
Fifth printing, March 1981
Sixth printing, June 1981
Seventh printing, November 1981
Eighth printing, March 1982
Ninth printing, July 1982
Tenth printing, October 1982
Eleventh printing, March 1983
Twelfth printing, July 1983
Thirteenth printing, December 1983
Fourteenth printing, April 1984
Fifteenth printing, November 1984
Sixteenth printing, August 1985
Seventeenth printing, December 1985
Eighteenth printing, April 1986
Nineteenth printing, December 1986
Twentieth printing, April 1987
Printed in the United States of America

Contents

Introduction

Today millions of people are discovering the benefits of movement. Everywhere you look they are out walking, jogging, running, playing tennis or racquetball, cycling or swimming. What do they hope to accomplish? Why this relatively sudden interest in physical fitness?

We are discovering that active people lead fuller lives. They have more stamina, resist illness, and stay trim. They have more self-confidence, are less depressed, and often, even late in life, are still working energetically at new projects.

In recent years, medical research has shown that a great deal of ill health is directly related to lack of physical activity. Awareness of this fact, along with fuller knowledge of health care, is changing lifestyles. The current enthusiasm for movement is not a fad. We now realize that the only way to prevent the diseases of inactivity is to remain active—not for a month, or a year, but for a lifetime.

Our ancestors did not have the problems that go with a sedentary life; they had to work hard to survive. They stayed strong and healthy through continuous, vigorous outdoor work: chopping, digging, tilling, planting, hunting, and all their other daily activities. But with the advent of the Industrial Revolution, machines began to do the work once done by hand. As people became less active, they began to lose strength and the instinct for natural movement.

Machines have obviously made life easier, but they have also created serious problems. Instead of walking, we drive; rather than climb stairs, we use elevators; while once we were almost continuously active, we now spend much of our lives sitting. Without daily physical exertion, our bodies become storehouses of unreleased tensions. With no natural outlets for our tensions, our muscles become weak and tight, and we lose touch with our physical nature, with life's energies.

But times are changing. The 1970's have brought us a critical awareness of the necessity for a healthy life. We have found that health is something we can control, that we can prevent poor health and disease. We are no longer content to sit and stagnate. Now, we are moving, rediscovering the joys of an active, healthy life. What's more, we can resume a more healthy and rewarding existence at any age.

The body's capacity for recovery is phenomenal. For example, a surgeon makes an incision, removes or corrects the problem, then sews you back up. At this point, the body takes over and heals itself. Nature finishes the surgeon's job. All of us have this seemingly miraculous capacity for regaining health, whether it be from something as drastic as surgery, or from poor physical condition caused by lack of activity and bad diet.

What does stretching have to do with all this? It is the important link between the sedentary life and the active life. It keeps the muscles supple, prepares you for movement, and helps you make the daily transition from inactivity to vigorous activity without undue strain. It is especially important if you run, cycle, play tennis or engage in other strenuous exercises, because activities like these promote tightness and inflexibility. Stretching before and after you work out will keep you flexible and help prevent common injuries such as shin splints or Achilles tendinitus from running, and sore shoulders or elbows from tennis.

With the tremendous number of people exercising now, the need for correct information is vital. Stretching is easy, but when it is done incorrectly, it can actually do more harm than good. For this reason it is essential to understand the right techniques.

For the past ten years I have worked with amateur and professional athletic teams and have participated in various sports medicine clinics throughout the country, and I have invariably found that few people (including professional athletes) know how to stretch correctly! I have been able to teach athletes that stretching is a simple, painless way of getting ready for movement. They have found it enjoyable and easy to do. And when they have stretched regularly and correctly, it has helped them to avoid injuries and perform to the best of their abilities.

Stretching feels good when done correctly. You do not have to push limits or attempt to go further each day. It should not be a personal contest to see how far you can stretch. Stretching should be tailored to your particular muscular structure, flexibility, and varying tension levels. The key is regularity and relaxation. The object is to reduce muscular tension, thereby promoting freer movement—not to concentrate on attaining extreme flexibility, which often leads to overstretching and injury.

We can learn a lot by observing animals. Watch a cat or a dog. They instinctively know how to stretch. They do so spontaneously, never overstretching, continually and naturally tuning up muscles they will have to use.

Stretching is not stressful. It is peaceful, relaxing and non-competitive. The subtle, invigorating feelings of stretching allow you to get in touch with your muscles. It is completely adjustable to the individual. You do not have to conform to any unyielding discipline; stretching gives you the freedom to be yourself and enjoy being yourself.

Anyone can be fit, with the right approach. You don't need to be a great athlete. But you do need to take it slowly, especially in the beginning. Give your body and mind time to adjust to the stresses of physical activity. Start easy and be regular. There is no way to get into shape in a day.

When you are stretching regularly and exercising frequently, you will learn to enjoy movement. Remember, each one of us is a unique physical and mental being with our own comfortable and enjoyable rhythms. We are all different in strength, endurance, flexibility and temperament. If you learn about your body and its needs, you will be able to develop your own personal potential and gradually build a foundation of fitness that will last a lifetime. □

Who Should Stretch

Everyone can learn to stretch, regardless of age or flexibility. You do not need to be in top physical condition or have specific athletic skills. Whether you sit at a desk all day, dig ditches, do housework, stand at an assembly line, drive a truck, or exercise regularly, the same techniques of stretching apply. The methods are gentle and easy, conforming to individual differences in muscle tension and flexibility. So, if you are healthy, without any specific physical problems, you can learn how to stretch safely and enjoyably.

Note:

Note: *If you have had any recent physical problems or surgery, particularly of the joints and muscles, or if you have been inactive or sedentary for some time, please consult your physician before you start a stretching or exercise program.*

When To Stretch

Stretching can be done any time you feel like it: at work, in a car, waiting for a bus, walking down the road, under a nice shady tree after a hike, or at the beach. Stretch before and after physical activity, but also stretch at various times of the day when you can. Here are some examples:

· In the morning before the start of the day.
· At work to release nervous tension.
· After sitting or standing for a long time.
· When you feel stiff.
· At odd times during the day, as for instance, when watching TV, listening to music, reading, or sitting and talking.

Why Stretch

Stretching, because it relaxes your mind and tunes up your body, should be part of your daily life. You will find that regular stretching will do the following things:

· Reduce muscle tension and make the body feel more relaxed.
· Help coordination by allowing for freer and easier movement.
· Increase range of motion.
· Prevent injuries such as muscle strains. (A strong, pre-stretched muscle resists stress better than a strong, unstretched muscle.)
· Make strenuous activities like running, skiing, tennis, swimming, cycling easier because it prepares you for activity; it's a way of signaling the muscles that they are about to be used.
· Develop body awareness. As you stretch various parts of the body, you focus on them and get in touch with them. You get to know yourself.
· Help loosen the mind's control of the body so that the body moves for "its own sake" rather than for competition or ego.
· Promote circulation.
· It feels good. □

How To Stretch

Stretching is easy to learn. But there is a right way and a wrong way to stretch. The right way is a relaxed, sustained stretch with your attention focused on the muscles being stretched. The wrong way (unfortunately practiced by many people), is to bounce up and down, or to stretch to the point of pain: these methods can actually do more harm than good.

If you stretch correctly and regularly, you will find that every movement you make becomes easier. It will take time to loosen up tight muscles or muscle groups, but time is quickly forgotten when you start to feel good.

The Easy Stretch

When you begin a stretch, spend 10-30 seconds in the *easy stretch*. No bouncing! Go to the point where you feel a *mild tension*, and relax as you hold the stretch. The feeling of tension should subside as you hold the position. If it does not, ease off slightly and find a degree of tension that is comfortable. The easy stretch reduces muscular tightness and readies the tissues for the developmental stretch.

The Developmental Stretch

After the easy stretch, move slowly into the *developmental stretch*. Again, no bouncing. Move a fraction of an inch further until you again feel a mild tension and hold for 10-30 seconds. Be in control. Again, the tension should diminish; if not, ease off slightly. The developmental stretch fine-tunes the muscles and increases flexibility.

Breathing

Your breathing should be slow, rhythmical and under control. If you are bending forward to do a stretch, exhale as you bend forward and then breathe slowly as you hold the stretch. Do not hold your breath while stretching. If a stretch position inhibits your natural breathing pattern, then you are obviously not relaxed. Just ease up on the stretch so you can breathe naturally.

Counting

At first, silently count the seconds for each stretch; this will insure that you hold the proper tension for a long enough time. After a while, you will be stretching by the way it feels, without the distraction of counting.

The Stretch Reflex

Your muscles are protected by a mechanism called the *stretch reflex*. Any time you stretch the muscle fibers too far (either by bouncing or overstretching), a nerve reflex responds by sending a signal to the muscles to contract; this keeps the muscles from being injured. Therefore, when you stretch too far, you tighten the very muscles you are trying to stretch! (You get a similar involuntary muscle reaction when you accidentally touch something hot; before you can think about it, your body quickly moves away from the heat.)

Holding a stretch as far as you can go or bouncing up and down strains the muscles and activates the stretch reflex. These harmful methods cause pain, as well as physical damage due to the microscopic tearing of muscle fibers. This tearing leads to the formation of scar tissue in the muscles, with a gradual loss of elasticity. The muscles become tight and sore. How can you get enthused about daily stretching and exercise when these potentially injurious methods are used?

Many of us were conditioned in high school to the idea of "no gain without pain." We learned to associate pain with physical improvement, and were taught that "...the more it hurts, the more you get out of it." But don't be fooled. Stretching, when done correctly, is not painful. Learn to pay attention to your body, for pain is an indication that something is *wrong*.

The easy and developmental stretches, as described on the previous page do not activate the stretch reflex and do not cause pain.

This Diagram Will Give You an Idea of a "Good Stretch":

← An Easy Stretch →	← The Developmental → Part of Stretching	← A Drastic Stretch →
(hold for 20-30 seconds)	*(hold for 30 seconds or longer)*	*(do not stretch in the drastic stretch)*

A STRETCH

The straight line diagram represents the stretch which is possible with your muscles and their connective tissue. You will find that your flexibility will naturally increase when you stretch, first in the easy, then in the developmental phase. By regularly stretching with comfortable and painless feelings you will be able to go beyond your present limits and come closer to your personal potential. □

Getting Started

After you have gone through these beginning stretches, you will start to develop a feeling for correct stretching. It is important to be aware of proper body alignment when stretching and to learn how to do each of the stretches in a way that is right for *your* body. Once you have learned how to stretch your body correctly, it is easy to learn and use the stretches in this book.

(Dotted areas indicate the parts of the body in which you will probably feel the stretch, but because no two people are the same, it is possible that you may feel a stretch in an area other than those marked.)

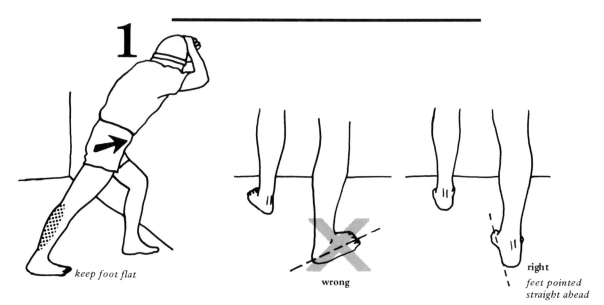

keep foot flat

wrong

right
*feet pointed
straight ahead*

Let's start with the calf stretch, a stretch for the back of the lower leg and ankle. Face a fence, wall, or something you can lean on for support. Stand a little distance from this support and rest your forearms on the support with your forehead on the back of your hands. Now bend one knee and bring it toward the support. The back leg should be straight with the foot flat and pointed straight ahead or slightly toed-in.

Now, without changing the position of your feet, slowly move your hips forward as you keep the back leg straight and your *foot flat*. Create an *easy feeling* of stretch in your calf muscle (*gastrocnemius*).

Hold an easy stretch for 20 seconds, then increase the stretch feeling very slightly into a developmental stretch for 20 seconds. Don't overstretch.

Now stretch the other calf. Does one leg feel different than the other? Is one leg more flexible than the other?

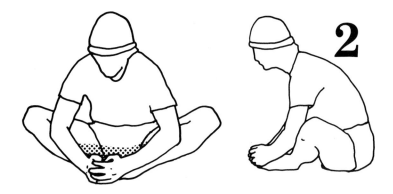

Sitting Groin Stretch: Next, sit on the floor. Put the soles of your feet together with your hands around your feet and toes. Be sure to keep your heels a comfortable distance from your crotch. Now gently pull your upper body forward until you feel an easy stretch in your groin area (inside of upper thighs). Hold an easy stretch for 20 seconds. If you are doing it right, it will feel good; the longer you hold the stretch, the less you should feel it. If possible, without strain, keep your elbows on the outside of your lower legs. This will help give the stretch position stability and balance.

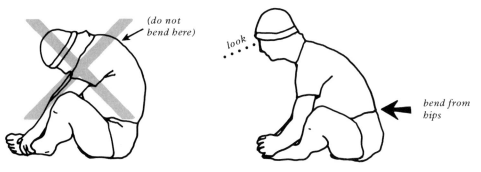

Do not initiate the movement forward from head and shoulders. This will round the shoulders and put pressure on lower back.

Be sure to concentrate on making the initial move forward from your hips. Keep your lower back flat. Look out in front of you.

After you feel the tension diminish slightly, increase the stretch by gently pulling yourself a little further into it. Now it should feel a bit more intense *but not painful*. Hold this for about 25 seconds. If the stretch is right in this developmental phase, the feeling of tension should slightly decrease or stay the same the longer the stretch is held, but it should not increase.

Slowly come out of the stretch. Please, no jerky, quick, bouncing movements! You must stop and hold each stretch so you can *really feel* what is happening with each position.

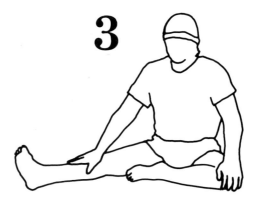

Next, straighten the right leg as you keep the left leg bent. The sole of the left foot should be facing the inside of the right upper leg. (Do not keep the knee of the straight leg "locked".) You are in a straight leg, bent knee position.

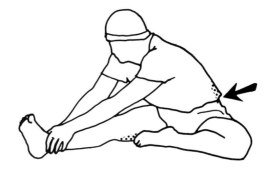

Now, to stretch the back of the upper right leg (hamstrings) and left side of the lower back (some will feel a stretch in the lower back, others won't), bend forward *from your hips* until the slightest, easiest feeling of stretch is created. Hold this easy stretch for 30 seconds. When you find what you think is the right stretch, touch the quadriceps of your right thigh to make sure that these muscles are relaxed. They should be spongy or soft, not tight or hard.

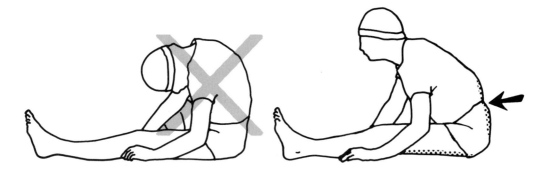

To find the stretch, do not make the initial movement with your head and shoulders. Do not try to touch your forehead to your knee. This will only encourage a backward tilt of the hips or pelvis and round your shoulders.

Be sure to initiate the stretch from the hips. Keep your chin in a neutral position (not held upward or downward). This will help keep the head and neck in a good position during the stretch. Keep shoulders and arms relaxed.

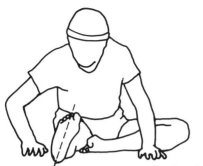

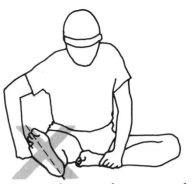

Be sure the foot of the leg being stretched is upright with ankle and toes relaxed. This will keep you a-ligned through ankle, knee, and hip.

Do not let your leg turn to the out-side because this causes misalign-ment of the leg and hip.

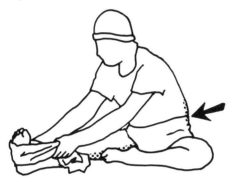

Use a towel, if necessary, around the bottom of your foot to help you do this stretch. If you are not very flexible the towel will help greatly in creat-ing and holding the right tension.

After the feeling of the easy stretch has subsided, slowly go into the develop-mental stretch. To find this developmental stretch you may only have to bend forward a fraction of an inch. Do not worry about how far you can go. A *very slight* distance in your bend forward may be all that is needed to reach the developmental phase. Remember, we are all different.

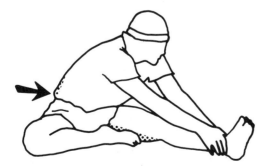

Now slowly come out of the stretch. Do the same stretch on the other side for left hamstring and right side of lower back. Remember to keep the front of your thigh relaxed and your foot upright with ankle and toes relaxed. First, do an easy stretch for 30 seconds, and then slowly find the develop-mental phase of the stretch and hold for 25 seconds. It takes time and per-sonal sensitivity to stretch properly.

Develop your ability to stretch by how you feel and not by how far you can stretch.

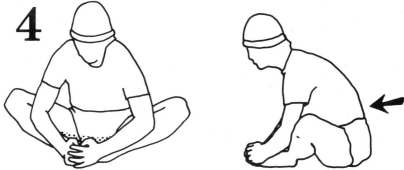

Repeat the sitting groin stretch. How does this feel as compared to the first time you did it? Any change at all?

A number of things are more important for you than concentrating solely on increasing flexibility:

1. Relaxation of tense areas such as feet, toes, hands, wrists, shoulders when stretching.
2. Learning how to find and control the right feeling of stretching.
3. Awareness of lower back, head and shoulders, and leg alignment during the stretch.
4. Adjusting to your changing body, for every day the body feels slightly different.

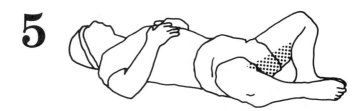

Lying Groin Stretch: Now lie on your back with the soles of your feet together. Let your knees fall apart. Relax your hips as you let gravity give you a very mild stretch in your groin area (inside of upper legs). Stay in this very relaxed position for 40 seconds. Really concentrate on letting go of any tension, do not force anything. The stretch feeling will be subtle and should happen naturally.

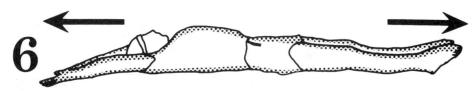

Slowly straighten both legs. With your arms overhead, reach with your arms and hands while you point your toes. This is an elongation stretch. Hold a controlled, good stretch for 5 seconds, then relax. Repeat 3 times. Each time you stretch, gently pull in your abdominal muscles to make the middle of your body thin. This feels really good. It stretches arms, shoulders, spine, abdominals, intercostal muscles of rib cage, feet, and ankles. This is an excellent, easy stretch to do first thing in the morning while still in bed.

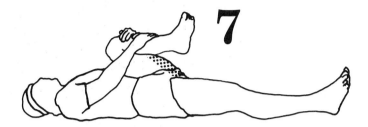

Next, bend one knee and gently pull it toward your chest until you feel an easy stretch. Hold for 40 seconds. You may feel a stretch in your lower back and back of the upper leg. If you do not feel any stretch, don't worry about it. This is an excellent position for the entire body, good for the lower back and very relaxing whether you feel a stretch or not. Do both sides and compare. Gradually get to know yourself.

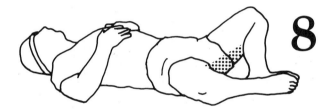

Repeat the lying groin stretch and just relax for 60 seconds. Let go of any tension in your feet, hands, and shoulders. You may want to do this stretch with your eyes closed.

How To Sit Up From A Lying Position:

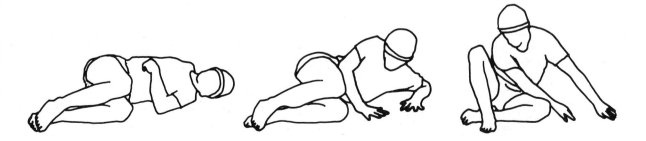

Bend both knees and roll over onto one side. While resting on your side, use your hands to push yourself up into a sitting position. By using your hands and arms this way, you take the pressure or stress off the back.

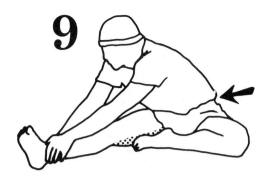

Now repeat the stretches for your hamstrings. Have you changed at all? Do you feel more limber and less tense than before stretching?

SUMMARY

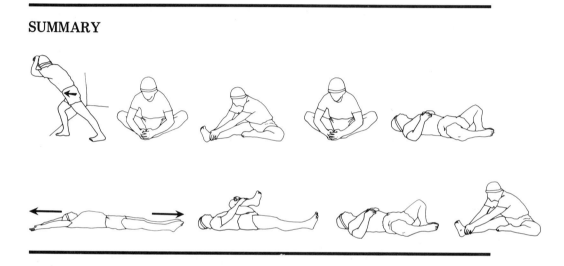

These are just a few stretches to get you started. I want you to understand that stretching is not a contest in flexibility. Your flexibility will naturally improve with proper stretching. Stretch with feelings you can enjoy. □

Many of the stretches should be held for 30-60 seconds. But after a while the time you hold stretches will vary. Sometimes you may want to hold one longer because you are extra tight that day, or you are just enjoying the stretch. *Remember that no two days are the same* so you must gauge your stretching by how you feel at the moment.

The Stretches

In the following section are the different stretches, with instructions for each position. They are presented as a series, but any of them may be done separately without doing the entire routine.

The drawings show the different positions, but you need not stretch as far as the drawings indicate. Stretch by how you feel without trying to imitate the figure in the drawings. Adjust each stretch to your own personal flexibility, which will vary daily.

Learn stretches for the various parts of your body, at first concentrating on the areas of greatest tension or tightness. On the following two pages is a guide to various muscles and body parts, with reference to the page where each may be found in the book.

Stretching Guide

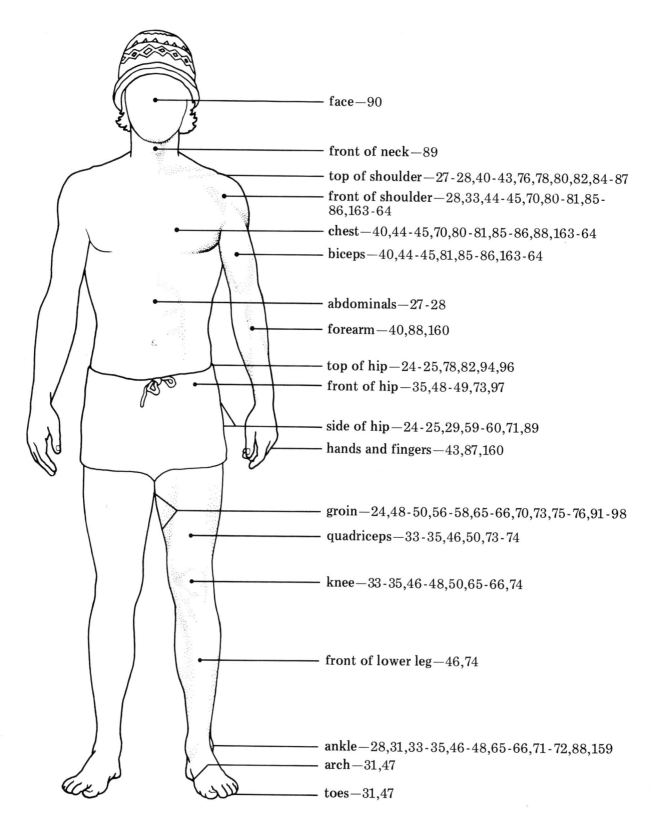

face—90

front of neck—89

top of shoulder—27-28,40-43,76,78,80,82,84-87

front of shoulder—28,33,44-45,70,80-81,85-86,163-64

chest—40,44-45,70,80-81,85-86,88,163-64

biceps—40,44-45,81,85-86,163-64

abdominals—27-28

forearm—40,88,160

top of hip—24-25,78,82,94,96

front of hip—35,48-49,73,97

side of hip—24-25,29,59-60,71,89

hands and fingers—43,87,160

groin—24,48-50,56-58,65-66,70,73,75-76,91-98

quadriceps—33-35,46,50,73-74

knee—33-35,46-48,50,65-66,74

front of lower leg—46,74

ankle—28,31,33-35,46-48,65-66,71-72,88,159

arch—31,47

toes—31,47

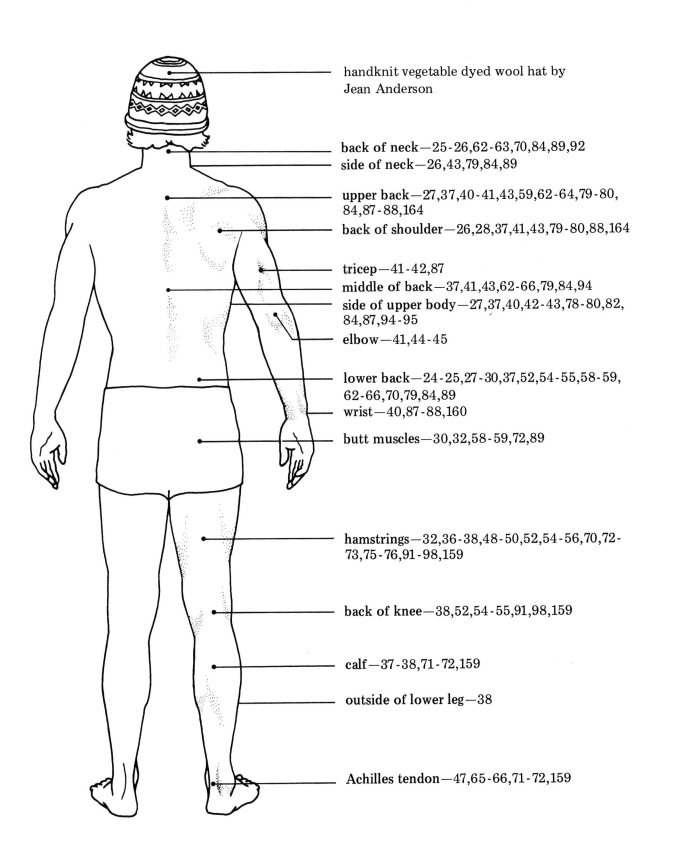

handknit vegetable dyed wool hat by
Jean Anderson

back of neck—25-26,62-63,70,84,89,92
side of neck—26,43,79,84,89

upper back—27,37,40-41,43,59,62-64,79-80,
84,87-88,164
back of shoulder—26,28,37,41,43,79-80,88,164

tricep—41-42,87
middle of back—37,41,43,62-66,79,84,94
side of upper body—27,37,40,42-43,78-80,82,
84,87,94-95
elbow—41,44-45

lower back—24-25,27-30,37,52,54-55,58-59,
62-66,70,79,84,89
wrist—40,87-88,160

butt muscles—30,32,58-59,72,89

hamstrings—32,36-38,48-50,52,54-56,70,72-
73,75-76,91-98,159

back of knee—38,52,54-55,91,98,159

calf—37-38,71-72,159

outside of lower leg—38

Achilles tendon—47,65-66,71-72,159

RELAXING STRETCHES FOR YOUR BACK

This is a short series of very easy stretches which you can do lying on your back. This series is beneficial because each position stretches a body area which is generally hard to relax. You can use this routine for mild stretching and relaxation.

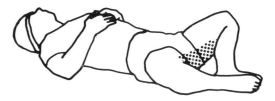

Relax, with knees bent and soles of your feet together. This comfortable position will stretch your groin. Hold for 30 seconds. Let the pull of gravity do the stretching.

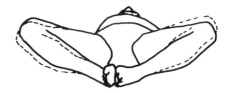

Variation: From this lying groin stretch, gently rock your legs as one unit (see illustration) back and forth about 10-12 times. These are real easy movements of no more than 1 inch in either direction. Initiate movements from top of hips. This will gently limber up your groin and hips.

A Stretch for the Lower Back, Side, and Top of Hip: The Secretary Stretch

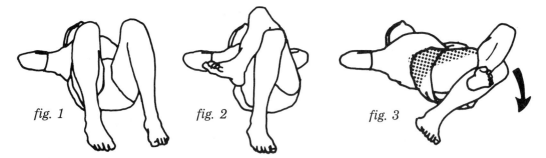

fig. 1   *fig. 2*   *fig. 3*

After gently stretching the groin, bring your knees together and rest your feet on the floor. Interlace your fingers behind your head and rest your arms on the floor (fig. 1). Now lift the left leg over the right leg (fig. 2). From here, use left leg to pull right leg toward floor (fig. 3) until you feel a good stretch along the side of the hip or in the lower back. Stretch and be relaxed. Keep the upper back, back of head, shoulders, and elbows flat on the floor. Hold for 30 seconds. *The idea is not to touch the floor with your right knee, but to stretch within* **your** *limits.* Repeat stretch for other side, crossing right over left leg and pulling down to the right.

This stretch position can be a real help if you have sciatic* problems of the lower back. If so, hold only stretch tensions that feel good. Never stretch to the point of pain.

Variation: Some people, especially women, will not feel a stretch. If that is the case with you, use opposite tension to create a stretch:

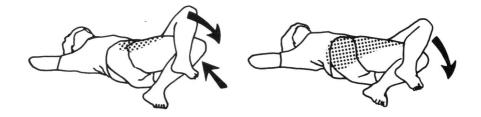

To do this, hold down the right leg with the left leg, as you try to pull the right leg back to an upright position (but, because you are holding the right leg down with the left leg, the right leg won't move). You will get a stretch on the side of the hip area. This technique is good for people who are tense as well as for those who are extremely limber in this area. A possible way to incorporate this variation in a series of stretches is to first do the regular secretary stretch (see p. 24), then use opposite tension, relax, and do the secretary stretch again.

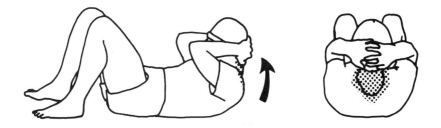

From the starting position of the last stretch for your back, you can stretch your upper spine and neck. This stretch helps reduce tension in the neck area and allows for freer movement of head and neck.

Interlace your fingers behind your head at about ear level. Now, use the power of your arms to slowly pull your head forward until you feel a slight stretch in the back of the neck. Hold for 5-10 seconds, then slowly return to the original starting position. Do this 3-4 times to gradually loosen up the upper spine and neck.

---

* The sciatic nerve is the longest and largest nerve of the body. It originates in the lumbar portion of the spine (lower back) and travels down the entire length of both legs and out to the great toe.

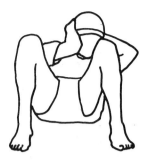

Variations: Gently pull your head and chin toward your left knee. Hold for 5 seconds. Relax and lower your head back down to the floor, then pull your head gently toward your right knee. Repeat 2-3 times.

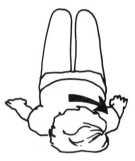

With the back of your head on the floor, turn your chin toward your shoulder (as you keep your head resting on the floor). Turn chin only as far as needed to get an easy stretch in the side of your neck. Hold 5 seconds, then stretch to the other side. Repeat 2-3 times.

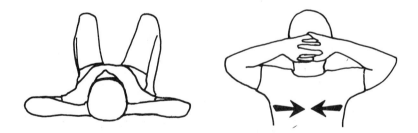

Shoulder Blade Pinch: From a bent-knee position, with your fingers interlaced behind your head, pull your shoulder blades together to create tension in the upper back area. (As you do this your chest should move upward.) Hold this controlled tension for 4-5 seconds., then relax and gently pull your head forward as shown on p. 25. This will help release tension and allow the neck to be stretched effectively.

Think of creating tension, relaxing the same area, then stretching the back of the neck to help keep the muscles of the neck free to move without tightness. Repeat 3-4 times.

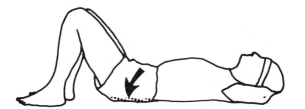

Lower Back Flattener: To relieve tension in lower back area, tighten your butt (*gluteus*) muscles and, at the same time, tighten your abdominal muscles to flatten your lower back. Hold this tension for 5-8 seconds, then relax. Repeat 2-3 times. Concentrate on maintaining constant muscle contraction. This pelvic tilting exercise will strengthen the butt and abdominal muscles so that you are able to sit and stand with good posture. Use these tension controls when sitting and standing.

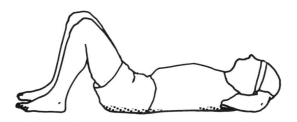

Shoulder Blade Pinch and Gluteus Tightener: Now, simultaneously do the shoulder blade pinch, flatten your lower back, and tighten your butt muscles. Hold 5 seconds, then relax and pull your head forward to stretch the back of your neck and upper back. Repeat 3-4 times. This feels real good.

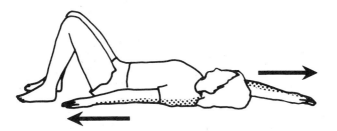

From a bent knee position, with your head resting on the floor, put one arm above your head (palm up) and the other arm down along your side (palm down). Now reach in opposite directions at the same time to create a controlled stretch in your shoulders and back. Hold stretch for 6-8 seconds. Do both sides at least twice. Keep your lower back relaxed and flat.

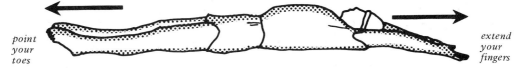

point your toes   *extend your fingers*

Elongation Stretch: Extend your arms overhead and straighten out your legs. Now reach as far as is comfortable in opposite direction with your arms and legs. Stretch for 5 seconds, and then relax.

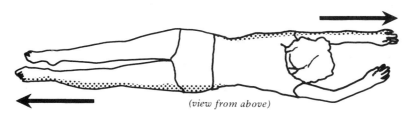

(view from above)

Now stretch diagonally. Point the toes of your left foot as you extend your right arm. Stretch as far as is comfortable. Hold 5 seconds, then relax. Stretch the right leg and the left arm the same way. Hold each stretch for at least 5 seconds, then relax.

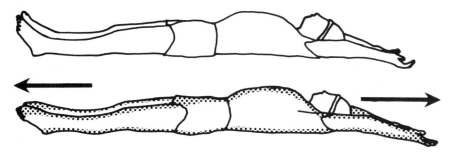

Now, at the same time, stretch both arms and both legs again. Hold 5 seconds, then relax. A good stretch for the muscles of the rib cage, abdominals, spine, shoulders, arms, ankles, and feet.

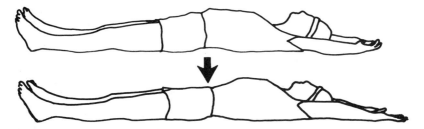

As a variation of this stretch, pull in with the abdominal muscles as you stretch. This will make you feel thin. Excellent exercise for your internal organs.

You may do these stretches as many times as you want. Usually three times is sufficient for reducing tension and tightness. These should help relax your spine and entire body. They help reduce overall body tension quickly. You could do these just before sleeping.

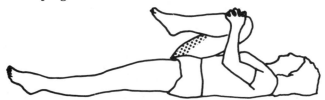

Pull your right leg toward your chest. For this stretch keep the back of your head on the floor or mat if possible, but don't strain. Hold an easy stretch for 30 seconds. Repeat, pulling your right leg toward your chest. Be sure to keep your lower back flat. If no real stretch is felt, don't worry. If the position feels good, use it. This is a very good position for the legs, feet, and back.

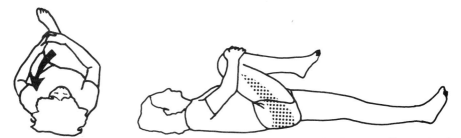

Variation: Pull your knee to your chest, then think of pulling the knee across your body toward your opposite shoulder to create a stretch on the outside of your right hip. Hold an easy stretch for 20 seconds. Do both sides.

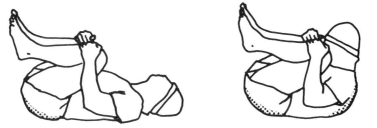

After pulling one leg at a time to your chest, pull both legs to your chest. This time concentrate on keeping the back of your head down and then curling your head up toward your knees.

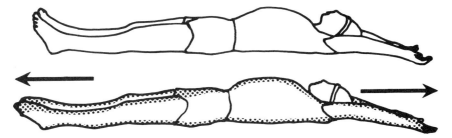

Again, straighten out both legs. Stretch and then relax.

A Stretch for the Lower Back and Side of Hip

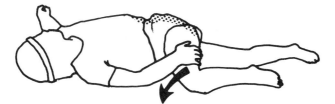

Bend one knee at 90° and, with your opposite hand, pull that bent leg up and over your other leg as shown above. Turn your head to look toward the hand of the arm that is straight (head should be resting on floor, not held up). Now, using the hand on your thigh (resting just above knee) pull your bent leg down toward the floor until you get the right stretch feeling in your lower back and side of hip. Keep feet and ankles relaxed. Make sure the back of your shoulders are flat on the floor. If not, the angle changes between the shoulders and the hips and it is more difficult to create a proper stretch. Hold an easy stretch for 30 seconds, each side.

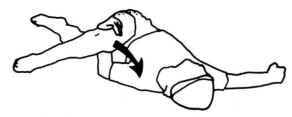

To increase the stretch in your buttocks, reach under your leg and behind your knee. Slowly pull knee toward opposite shoulder until you get the right stretch. Keep both shoulders flat on floor. Hold for 15-25 seconds.

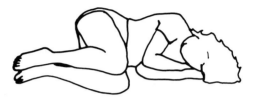

You can end a series of stretches for your back by lying in the "fetus position." Lie on your side with your legs curled up and your head resting on your hands. Relax.

SUMMARY

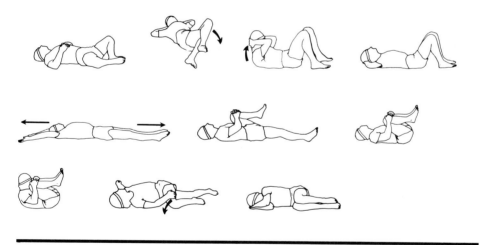

Learn to listen to your body. If the tension builds or you feel pain, your body is trying to let you know that something is wrong, that there is a problem. If this happens, ease off slightly until the stretch *feels* right.

STRETCHES FOR THE LEGS, FEET, AND ANKLES

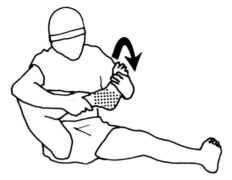

Rotate your ankle clockwise and counter-clockwise through a complete range of motion with slight resistance provided by your hand. Rotary motion of the ankle helps to gently stretch out tight ligaments. Repeat 10-20 times in each direction. Do this to both ankles and feel if there is any difference between ankles in terms of tightness and range of motion. Sometimes an ankle that has been sprained will feel a bit weaker and tighter. This difference may go unnoticed until you work each ankle separately and compare.

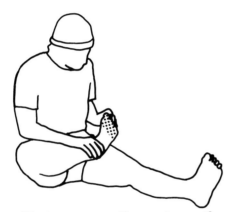

Next, use your fingers to gently pull the toes toward you to stretch the top of the foot and tendons of the toes. Hold an easy stretch for 10 seconds. Repeat 2-3 times.

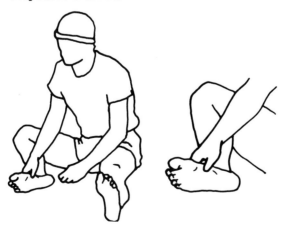

With your thumbs, massage up and down the longitudinal arch of your foot. Use circular motions with a good amount of pressure to loosen tissues. Do both feet. Can you feel any tenseness or tightness? Always massage each arch

2-3 minutes before bedtime. It will relax your feet. This is good to do spontaneously while watching TV, or just before going to sleep. Massage with a pressure that feels good.

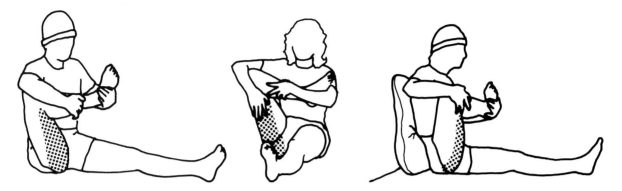

To stretch the upper hamstrings and hip, hold onto the outside of your ankle with one hand, with your other hand and forearm around your bent knee. Gently pull the leg *as one unit* toward your chest until you feel an easy stretch in the back of the upper leg. You may want to do this stretch while you rest your back against something for support. Hold 20 seconds. Make sure the leg is pulled as one unit so no stress is felt in the knee. After this, slightly increase the stretch by pulling the leg a little closer to your chest. Hold this developmental stretch for 20 seconds. Do both sides. Is one leg more flexible than the other?

For some of you, this position will not provide a stretch. If that is the case, do the stretch shown below.

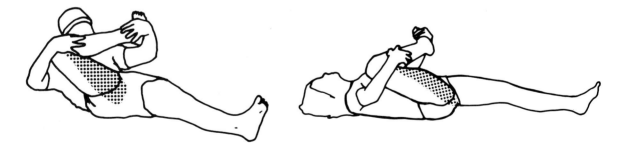

Begin this stretch lying down, then lean forward to hold on to your leg as described in the previous stretch. Gently pull leg as one unit toward your chest until you feel an easy stretch in the butt and upper hamstring. Hold for 20 seconds. Doing this stretch in a lying position will increase the stretch in the hamstrings for people who are relatively flexible in this area. Do both legs and compare.

Experiment: see the difference in the stretch when your head is forward and when the back of your head is on the floor. Always keep every stretch within a personal comfort range.

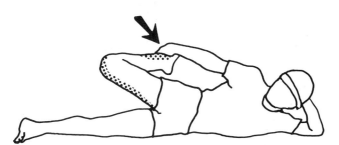

Lie on your left side and rest the side of your head in the palm of your left hand. Hold the top of your right foot with your right hand between the toes and ankle joint. Gently pull the right heel toward the right buttock to stretch the ankle and quadriceps (front of thigh). Hold an easy stretch for 10 seconds. *Never stretch the knee to the point of pain. Always be in control.*

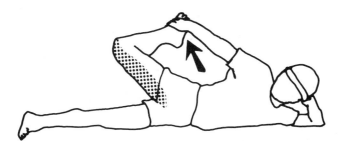

Now move the front of your right hip forward by contracting the right butt (*gluteus*) muscles as you push your right foot into your right hand. This should stretch the front of your thigh. Hold an easy stretch for 10 seconds. Keep the body in a straight line. Now stretch the left leg in the same way. You may get a good stretch in the front of the shoulder. At first it may be hard to hold this for very long. Just work on the proper way to stretch without worrying about flexibility or how you look. Regularity with stretching will create a positive change.

If you experience any knee problems with these stretches, don't do them. Instead, use the opposite-hand-to-opposite-foot technique of stretching the knee (p. 74).

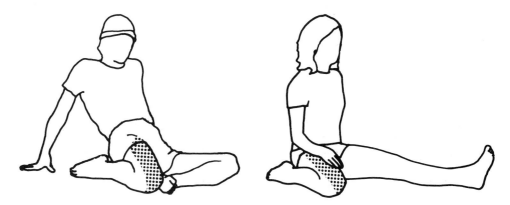

A Sitting Stretch for the Quadriceps: First sit with your right leg bent, with your right heel just to the outside of your right hip. The left leg is bent and the sole of your left foot is next to the inside of your upper right leg. (You could also do this stretch with your left leg straight out in front of you.)

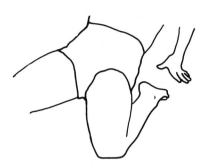
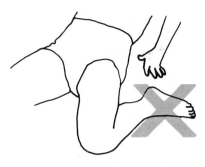

In this stretch position your foot should be extended back with the ankle flexed. If your ankle is tight and restricts the stretch, move your foot just enough to the side to lessen the tension in your ankle.

Try not to let your foot flare out to the side in this position. By keeping your foot pointed straight back you take the stress off the inside of your knee. The more your foot flares to the side, the more stress there is on your knee.

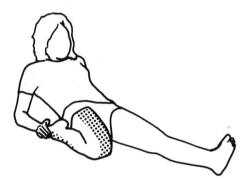

Now, slowly lean *straight back* until you feel an easy stretch. Use your hands for balance and support. Hold this easy stretch for 30 seconds.

Some people will have to lean back a lot further than others to find the right stretch tension. And some people may feel the right stretch without leaning back at all. Just be aware of how you feel and forget about how far you can go. Get into what *you* can do and don't worry about anyone else.

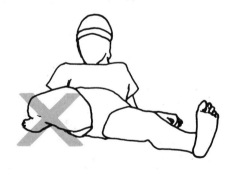

Do not let your knee lift off the floor or mat. If your knee comes up you are overstretching by leaning back too far. Ease up on the stretch.

Now slowly, and with complete control, increase into the developmental stretch. Hold for 25 seconds, then slowly come out of it. Switch sides and stretch the left thigh the same way.

Can you feel any difference in tension in the two stretches? Is one side more limber than the other? Are you more flexible on one side?

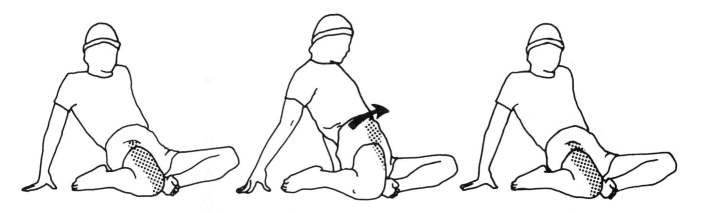

After stretching your quads, practice tightening the buttocks on the side of the bent leg as you turn the hip over. This will help stretch the front of your hip and give a better overall stretch to upper thigh area. After contracting the butt muscles for 5-8 seconds, let the buttocks relax. Drop your hip down and continue to stretch the quad for another 15 seconds. Practice to eventually get both sides of the buttocks to touch the floor at the same time during the quad stretch. Now do other side.

Note: Stretching the quad first, then turning the hip over as the buttocks contract will help change the stretch feeling when you return to the original quad stretch.

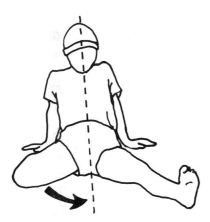 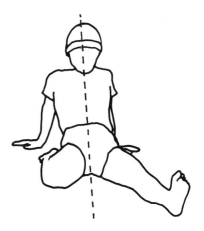

If, during the stretch, there is any pain in the knee joint, move the knee of the leg being stretched closer to the midline of your body and see if you can find a more comfortable position.

Moving your knee closer to the midline of your body may take the stress off of the knee, but *if there is pain which does not subside in any variation of this position, discontinue doing this particular stretch.*

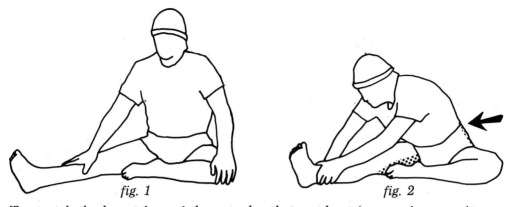

fig. 1   *fig. 2*

To stretch the hamstrings of the same leg that was bent (see previous page), straighten the right leg with the sole of your left foot slightly touching the inside of the right thigh. You are now in the straight-leg, bent-knee position (fig. 1). Slowly bend forward from the hips toward the foot of the straight leg (fig. 2) until you create the slightest feeling of stretch. Hold this for 20 seconds. After the stretch feeling has diminished, bend a bit more forward from the hips. Hold this developmental stretch for 25 seconds. Then switch sides and stretch the left leg in the same manner.

During this stretch, keep the foot of the straight leg upright with the ankle and toes relaxed. Be sure the quadriceps are soft to the touch (relaxed) during the stretch. Do not dip your head forward when initiating the stretch (see pp. 16-17, *Getting Started*).

I have found that it is best to first stretch your quads, then the hamstrings of the same leg. It is easier to stretch the hamstrings after the quadriceps have been stretched.

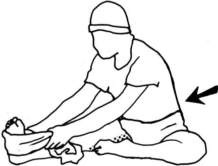

Use a towel to help you stretch if you cannot *easily* reach your feet.

Get used to doing variations of basic stretches. In each variation you will use your body in a different way. You will become more aware of all the stretch possibilities when you change the angles of the stretch tension, even if the angle changes are very slight.

Variations of the Straight-leg, Bent-knee Position:

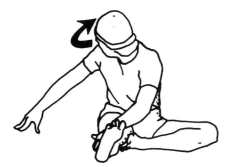

Reach across your body with your left arm to the outside of your right leg. Place your right hand out to the side for balance. This will stretch the muscles of the upper back and spine and the side of the lower back, as well as the hamstrings. To change the stretch, look over your right shoulder as you slightly turn the front of your left hip to the inside. This will stretch the lower back and in between the shoulder blades.

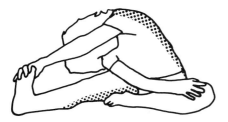

If you are especially flexible, you can increase the stretch along your sides with a variation of this position: with your right leg straight, reach over your head with your left arm and grab the outside of your right foot. As you bend, rest your right hand on your left knee. This is an excellent stretch for the hamstrings and the lateral portion of the upper body. It helps keep the waistline trim.

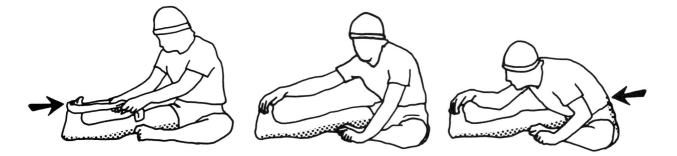

To stretch the back of the lower leg (calf and soleus muscles), either use a towel around the ball of your foot to pull your toes toward your knee, or if you are more flexible, use your hand to pull your toes toward your knee. Find an easy stretch and hold for 25 seconds. You may need to lean forward at the waist (from the hips) to increase the stretch.

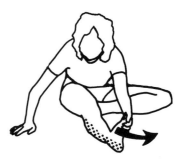

To stretch the outside of your lower leg, reach down with your opposite hand and hold on to the outside border of your foot (see drawing). Now, gently turn the outside of the foot to the inside to feel a stretch in the outside of the lower leg. This stretch should be done with a straight leg, but the leg should be bent if you are unable to *easily* hold on to the outside border of your foot with your leg straight. In this straight-leg position the quadriceps should be soft, relaxed. Hold an easy stretch for 25 seconds.

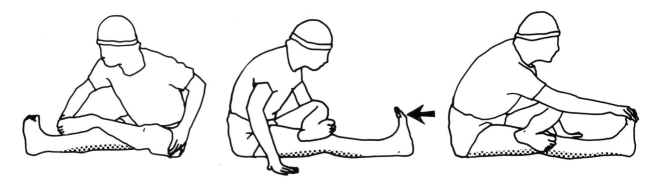

To isolate a stretch in the back of the knee, start with one leg straight. Then bend the other knee, and set the bent leg on top of the straight leg with the ankle of the bent leg resting just to the outside of the other leg and just above (*not on*) the knee. Now gently bend forward from your hips until an easy tension is felt behind your knee. Hold the easy stretch for 20 seconds and the developmental stretch for 15 seconds. This is very good for people who are tight behind the knee. But always be aware of overstretching.

Never lock your knees when doing sitting stretches. Be sure to keep the front of your thigh (quadriceps) relaxed in all positions using a straight leg. It is impossible to stretch the hamstrings correctly when the opposing set of muscles, the quadriceps, are not relaxed.

SUMMARY

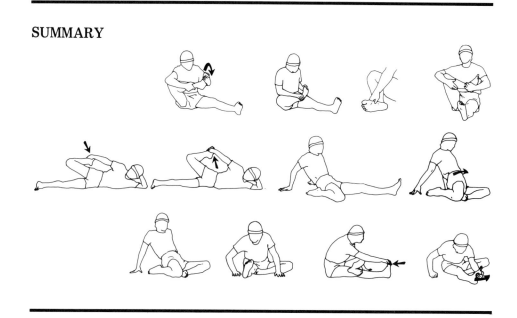

Bouncing movements while stretching can actually make you tighter rather than more flexible. For example, if you bounce four or five times while touching your toes (which most of us did in high school), then several minutes later bend over again, you will probably find that you are farther away from your toes than when you started! Each bouncing movement activates the stretch reflex, tightening the very muscles you are trying to stretch.

STRETCHES FOR THE BACK, SHOULDERS, AND ARMS:

Many people suffer from tension in the upper body because of the mental stress of modern living. Quite a few muscular athletes are stiff in the upper body because of not stretching that area.

There are many stretches that can reduce tension and increase flexibility in the upper body. Most of them can be done anywhere.

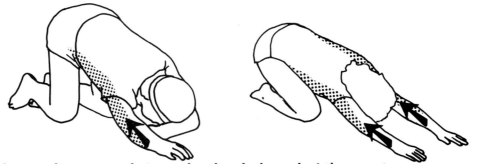

With legs bent under you, reach forward and grab the end of the carpet or mat. If you can't grab on to something, just pull back with straight arms while you press down slightly with your palms.

You can do this stretch one arm at a time or both at the same time. Pulling with just one arm provides more control and isolates the stretch on either side. You should feel this in your shoulders, arms, lats (*latissimus dorsi*) or sides, upper back, and even your lower back. When you do this for the first time you may only feel it in the shoulders and arms, but as you do it more you will learn to stretch other areas. By slightly moving your hips in either direction you can increase or decrease the stretch. Don't strain. Be relaxed. Hold for 15 seconds.

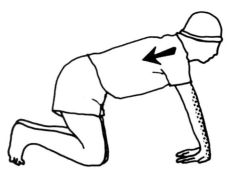

A Forearm and Wrist Stretch: Start on all fours. Support yourself on your hands and knees. Thumbs should be pointed to the outside with fingers pointed toward knees. Keep palms flat as you lean back to stretch the front part of your forearms. Hold an easy stretch for 20 seconds. Relax, then stretch again. You may find you are very tight in this area.

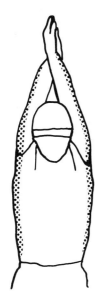

With arms extended overhead and palms together as drawing shows, stretch arms upward and slightly backwards. Breathe in as you stretch upward, holding the stretch for 5-8 seconds.

This is a great stretch for the muscles of the outer portions of the arms, shoulders, and ribs. It can be done any time and any place to relieve tension and create a feeling of relaxation and well-being.

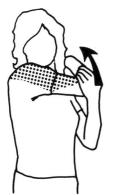

To stretch your shoulder and middle of upper back, gently pull your elbow across your chest toward your opposite shoulder. Hold stretch for 10 seconds.

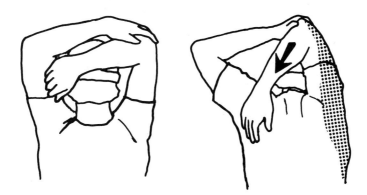

Here is a simple stretch for your triceps and the top of your shoulders. With arms overhead, hold the elbow of one arm with the hand of the other arm. Gently pull the elbow behind your head, creating a stretch. Do it slowly. Hold for 15 seconds. Do not use drastic force to limber up.

Stretch both sides. Does it feel like one side is a lot tighter than the other side? This is a good way to begin loosening up your arms and shoulders. You can do this stretch while walking.

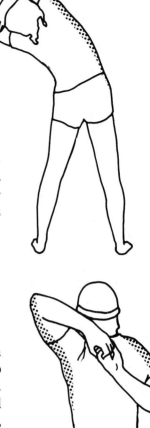

Variation: From a standing position, with your knees slightly bent (1 inch), gently pull your elbow behind your head as you bend from your hips to the side. Hold an easy stretch for 10 seconds. Do both sides. Keeping your knees slightly bent will give you better balance while you stretch.

Another Shoulder Stretch: Reach behind your head and down as far as you can with your left hand and, if you are able, grab your right hand coming up, palm out. Grab fingers and hold. Many will not be able to do this stretch without help. Hold only as long as fairly comfortable. If your hands do not meet, try one of these:

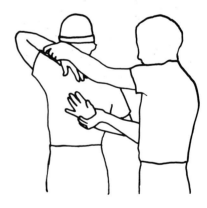

Have someone pull your hands slowly toward each other until you get an easy stretch and hold it. Do not stretch too far. You may get a great stretch without having your fingers touching. Stretch within *your* limits.

OR

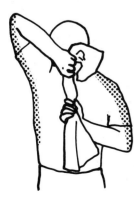

Drop a towel behind your head. With your upper arm bent, reach up with your other arm to hold on to the end of the towel. Gradually move your hand up on the towel, pulling your upper arm down, until your hands are touching.

Work a little on it every day and get a good stretch. After a while you will be able to do this stretch without help. It reduces tension and increases flexibility. It also acts as an upper body revitalizer when you are tired.

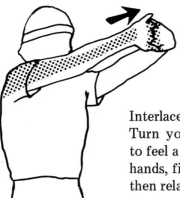

Interlace your fingers out in front of you at shoulder height. Turn your palms outward as you extend your arms forward to feel a stretch in your shoulders, middle of upper back, arms, hands, fingers, and wrists. Hold an easy stretch for 15 seconds, then relax and repeat.

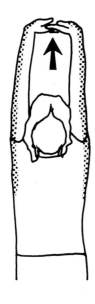

Interlace your fingers above your head. Now, with your palms facing upward, push your arms slightly back and up. Feel the stretch in arms, shoulders, and upper back. Hold stretch for 15 seconds. Do not hold your breath. This stretch is good to do anywhere, anytime. Excellent for slumping shoulders.

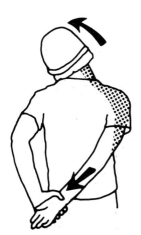

To stretch the side of your neck and top of shoulder, lean your head sideways toward your left shoulder as your left hand pulls your right arm down and across, behind your back. Hold an easy stretch for 10 seconds. Do both sides. This stretch can be done sitting on the floor, in a chair, or while standing.

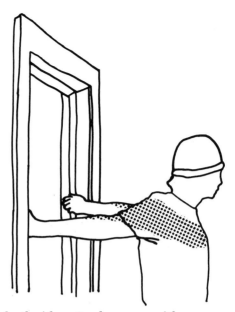

Another stretch is to hold on to a fence or both sides of a doorway with your hands behind you at about shoulder level. Let your arms straighten as you lean forward. Hold your chest up and chin in.

The next stretches are done with your fingers interlaced behind your back.

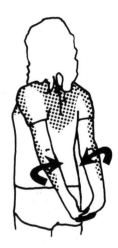

For the first stretch, slowly turn your elbows inward while straightening your arms.

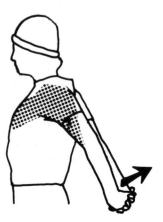

If that is fairly easy, then lift your arms up behind you until you feel a stretch in the arms, shoulders or chest. Hold an easy stretch for 5-15 seconds. This is good to do when you find yourself slumping forward from the shoulders. Keep your chest out and chin in. This stretch can be done any time.

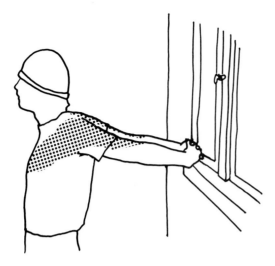

To further stretch your chest and shoulders, bring your arms up behind you, keeping your arms and back straight, without tilting forward. Rest your hands on something for support. As you take a few steps away from the object and straighten your arms you will increase the stretch. *Do not overstretch.* This is great for rounded shoulders and gives an immediate feeling of energy.

SUMMARY

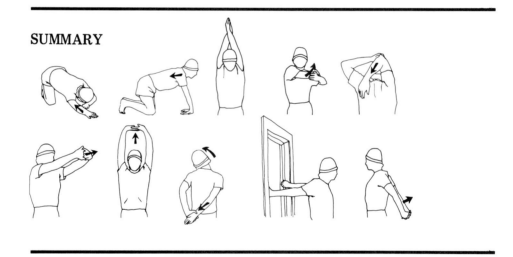

It is better to understretch than to overstretch. Always be at a point where you can stretch further, and never at a point where you have gone as far as you can go.

A SERIES OF STRETCHES FOR THE LEGS

Toe Pointer: This is another good stretch for the legs. You can do a series of stretches for the legs, feet, and groin from the toe pointer position:

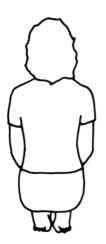 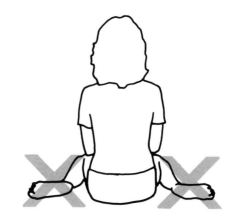

This position helps stretch the knees, ankles, and quadriceps. The toe pointer will also help relax the calves so they may be stretched more easily.

Do not let your feet flare out to the sides when doing this stretch. A flared-out position of the lower legs and feet may cause overstretching of the inside (medial collateral) ligaments of the knee.

Caution: *If you have or have had knee problems be very careful bending the knees underneath you. Do it slowly and under control.*

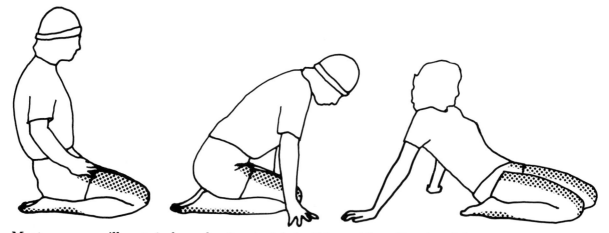

Most women will not feel much of a stretch in this position. But for tight people, especially men, this lets you know if you have tight ankles. If there is a strain, place your hands on the outside of your legs for support as you balance yourself slightly forward. Find a position you can hold for 20-30 seconds.

If you are tight, do not overstretch. Regularity with stretching creates positive change. There will be noticeable improvement in ankle flexibility within several weeks.

Variation:

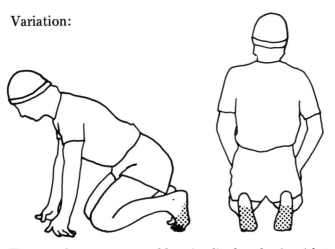

To stretch your toes and longitudinal arch, sit with toes underneath you (see above). Put your hands in front of you for balance and control. If more stretch is desired, slowly lean backwards until it feels right. Hold only stretches that feel good and you can control. Stretch easily for 15 seconds. Be careful. There may be a lot of tension in this part of the foot and toes. Have patience with yourself. Gradually get your body used to changing by regular stretching. Then return to toe pointer after doing this stretch.

To Stretch the Achilles Tendons and Ankles:

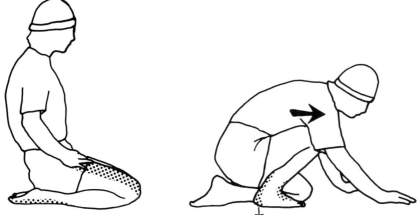

Bring the toes of one foot almost even or parallel to the knee of the other leg. Let the heel of the bent leg come off the ground one-half inch or so. Lower heel toward ground while pushing forward on your thigh (just above the knee) with your chest and shoulder. The idea is not to get the heel flat but to use the forward pressure from your shoulder on your thigh to give an easy stretch to the Achilles tendon. All that is needed to adequately stretch the Achilles tendon is a *very slight stretch*. Hold 15 seconds.

This stretch is great for tight ankles and arches. Be sure to work both sides. Here again, you will probably find that one side is a lot different than the other in flexibility and feeling. As we get older or go through periods of inactivity and then are active again, there is a lot of stress and strain on the ankles and arches. One way to reduce or eliminate the pain and soreness of new activity is to stretch before and after exercise.

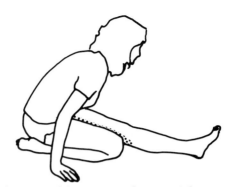

To stretch the hamstrings from the toe pointer position, extend or straighten one leg out in front of you, with the heel of that forward foot resting on the floor and the other leg still bent under you. *Be sure to use your arms and hands for balance and support* so you don't have too much pressure on the leg you are sitting on, nor too much of a stretch in the hamstrings you are stretching. *This is an advanced stretch for the hamstrings.* It intensifies the stretch in the straight leg. Gently bend forward from the waist until you feel an easy stretch. Hold for 20 seconds. Keep your butt close to the heel of the bent leg. Stretch within your comfortable limits.

Be careful if you have or have had knee problems. Do not stretch with any feeling of actual pain. Learn how to control yourself so the proper stretch feeling can be found.

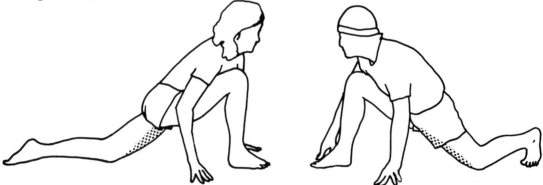

To stretch the muscles in the front of the hip (*iliopsoas*), move one leg forward until the knee of the forward leg is directly over the ankle. Your other knee should be resting on the floor. Now, without changing the position of the knee on the floor or the forward foot, lower the front of your hip downward to create an easy stretch. Hold for 30 seconds. You should feel this stretch in the front of the hip and possibly in the hamstrings and groin. This is excellent for lower back problems.

Stretching for 10-30 minutes in the evening is a good way to keep your muscles well tuned, so you feel good the next morning. If you have any tight areas, or soreness, stretch these areas before retiring and feel for yourself the difference the next morning.

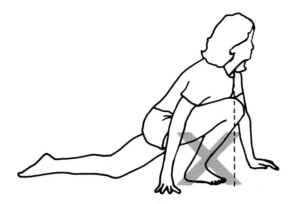

Do not have your knee forward of the ankle. This will hinder the proper stretching of the hip and legs. The greater distance there is between the back knee and the heel of the front foot, the easier it is to stretch the hip and legs.

Variations:

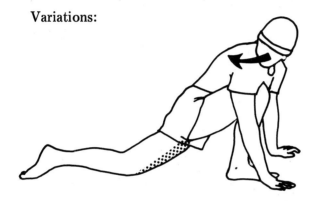

Turn the left hip slowly to the inside to change the area of the stretch. By only slightly changing the angles of stretch you are able to stretch many different, adjacent areas of the body. Hold an easy stretch for 20 seconds. This is excellent for hips, lower back, and groin. Also, get used to looking over your shoulder, behind you, to add a further stretch to the position.

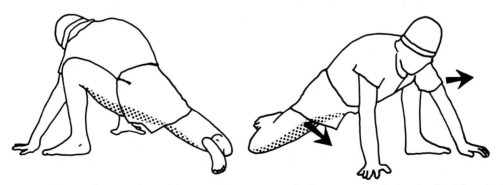

From the previous hip stretch you can isolate a stretch in the inside of the upper leg. Bend your rear knee and move your rear foot to the inside. This will make a 90° angle at the knee joint. Now move your shoulders off your knee and put your hands to the inside of your body for support. Move hips downward to stretch the inside of your upper leg (groin). Do not move your back knee or front foot. Be sure that your front knee is directly above your ankle. Hold an easy stretch for 25 seconds.

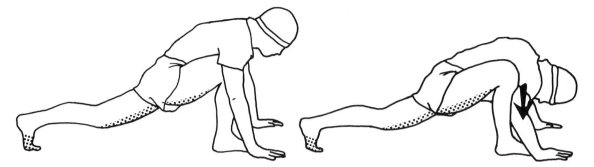

With your front knee directly above your ankle, shift your weight up onto the toes and ball of your back foot. Now hold an easy stretch with a fairly straight back leg for 20 seconds. Think of the front of your hip going down to create the right stretch tension. Use hands for balance. This stretches the groin, hamstrings, and hip, and possibly behind the knee of the back leg. Hold 15 seconds. Do both legs. An excellent stretch for hip flexibility.

Another variation is to change the stretch by gently lowering your upper body to the inside of the knee of the forward leg. Hold a comfortable stretch for 20 seconds.

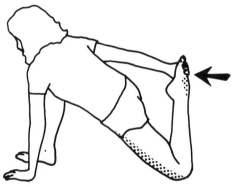

To stretch the quadricep muscle, reach behind you with your right hand and grab the top of your left foot between your ankle and toes. Now slowly lower the front of your hip downward as you gently pull your left heel toward the middle of your buttocks until you feel a slight stretch. Hold an easy stretch 20 seconds. A great position to isolate a stretch in. *Be careful if you have had knee problems.*

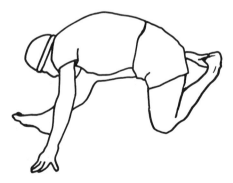

If you cannot easily reach your foot, move your hips back without changing the position of your front foot and back knee. Lean back and grab the top of your foot with your opposite hand, then move your hips slightly forward and downward as you pull your heel to the middle of your buttocks. You may need to move only an inch or two forward to create a feeling of stretch. Hold a slight stretch for 15 seconds. Be careful not to overstretch as you lean forward.

SUMMARY

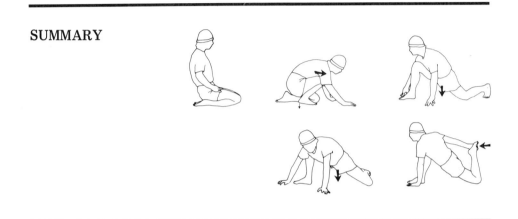

You would think we would know a great deal about staying in shape from the thousands of hours invested in high school P.E. classes. Yet most of us learned only games and sports. Ask yourself: What do I do in my daily living that I enjoy and was taught in school? It's amazing to think how little we learned in all those hours. We could have learned how to take care of ourselves, how to keep from becoming old before our time, and how to avoid suffering from back problems brought about by bad habits. But now we are teaching ourselves what we should have learned in school; and we haven't started any too soon.

STRETCHES FOR THE LOWER BACK, HIPS, GROIN & HAMSTRINGS

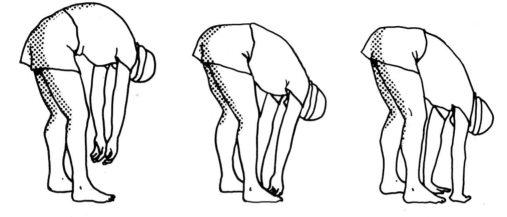

Start in a standing position with feet about shoulder-width apart and pointed straight ahead. Slowly bend forward from the hips. Always keep knees slightly bent during the stretch (1 inch) so lower back is not stressed. Let your neck and arms relax. Go to the point where you feel a slight stretch in the back of your legs. Stretch in this easy phase for 15-25 seconds, until you are relaxed. Let yourself relax physically by mentally concentrating on the area being stretched. Do not stretch with knees locked or bounce when you stretch. Simply hold an easy stretch. Stretch by how you feel and not by how far you can go.

When you do this stretch you will feel it mostly in the hamstrings (back of thighs) and back of the knees. The back will also be stretched, but most of the stretch will be felt in the back of the legs.

Some of you will be able to touch your toes, or just above the ankles. Although we are different in flexibility, we do have one thing in common: we are all stretching our muscles.

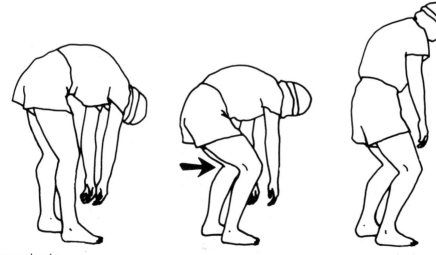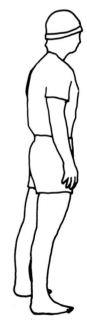

Important:
Any time you bend at the waist to stretch, remember to bend your knees

slightly (1 inch or so). It takes the pressure off your lower back. Use the big muscles of the upper legs to stand up, instead of the small muscles of the lower back. Never bring yourself to an upright position with knees locked.

This is a particularly good stretch to do before any kind of heavy labor, especially in the morning or when weather is cold. By protecting the muscles in the lower back, many injuries will be prevented.

This principle is important in lifting heavy objects off the ground (see p. 106).

Next, assume a bent-knee position with your heels flat, toes pointed straight ahead and feet about shoulder-width apart. Hold this position for 30 seconds.

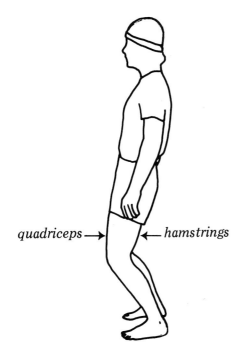

quadriceps → ← hamstrings

In this bent-knee position you are tightening the quadriceps and relaxing the hamstrings. The primary function of the quadriceps is to straighten the leg. The basic function of the hamstrings is to bend the knee. Because these muscles have opposing actions, tightening the quadriceps will relax the hamstrings.

Now, as you hold this bent-knee position, feel the difference between the front of the thigh and the back of the thigh. The quadriceps should feel hard and tight while the hamstrings should feel soft and relaxed. It is easier to stretch the hamstrings if they have been relaxed first.

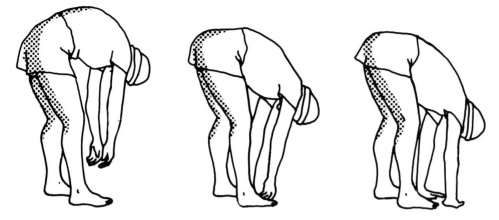

After holding the bent-knee position, stand up and then bend down again with knees slightly bent (1 inch, see p. 52): don't bounce. You probably can go a little farther already. Hold this stretch for about 30 seconds.

A reminder: bend your knees when you stand up.

You must be in a comfortable and stable position when you stretch.

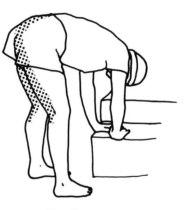

You will find it easier to hold this stretch if you can distribute your weight between your arms and legs. If you are unable to rest your palms on the ground with your knees slightly bent (many people cannot), then use a stair or curb, or a pile of books to rest your hands on. Find an even, light stretch. Find a balance between your hands and feet so you can relax.

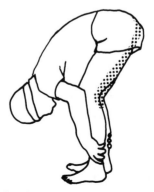

Another variation of this stretch is to hold onto the back of your lower legs in the calf or ankle area with your hands. By pulling your upper body downward with your hands you will be able to increase the stretch in your legs and back, while you concentrate on relaxing in a very stable position. Do not go too far. Pull yourself down only to where you can be relaxed. Stretch and hold. Keep your knees slightly bent.

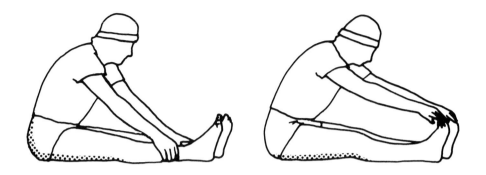

Next, sit down with your legs straight and feet upright, heels no more than six inches apart. Bend from the hips to get an easy stretch. Hold for 20 seconds. You will probably feel this just behind the knees, and in the back of the upper legs. You may also feel a stretch in the lower back if your back is tight.

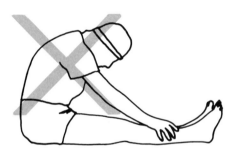

Do not dip your head forward as you begin this stretch. Try to keep your hips from rolling backwards.

Think of bending from your hips without rounding your lower back.

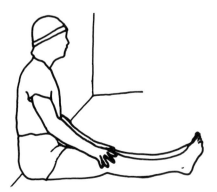

You may need to sit against a wall to keep your lower back flat. This position in itself may be enough of a stretch for you if you are extremely tight.

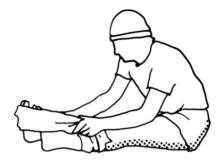

If you have trouble finding a place where you can stretch and relax, then use a towel to help. Place the towel around your feet, grab it by the ends and pull yourself forward from the hips to where you can relax and still get a stretch. Use straight arms to pull yourself forward. Work your way down the towel with your fingers, until the stretch feels right.

If this stretch seems to put pressure on your lower back or you have had lower back problems, do the stretches shown on page 36. This will feel more comfortable.

Be careful when you stretch with both legs in front of you or when bending forward at the hips in a standing position. You must not overstretch in these positions. Since the back of each leg probably differs in tightness and tension, stretching both legs at the same time should be avoided if you have lower back problems. When one or both legs are extremely tight, it is difficult to stretch both legs at the same time and get the correct stretch for each leg. It is easier on your back to stretch each leg separately.

To Stretch the Groin Area

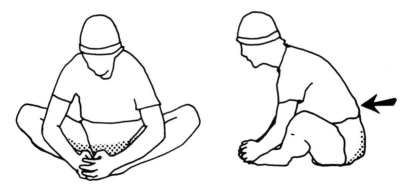

Put the soles of your feet together and hold onto your toes. Gently pull yourself forward, bending from the hips, until you feel a good stretch in your groin. You may also feel a stretch in the back. Hold for 40 seconds. Do not make initial movement for stretch from head and shoulders. Move from the hips (see p. 15, *Getting Started*). Try to get your elbows on the outside of your legs so the stretch position has stability and balance. It is easier to stretch when you are perfectly stable.

Remember—no bouncing when you stretch. Find a place that is fairly comfortable that allows you to stretch and relax at the same time.

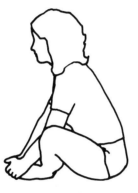

If you have any trouble bending forward, perhaps your heels are too close to your groin area.

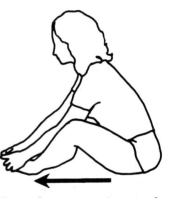

If so, keep your feet farther out in front of you. This will allow you to get movement forward.

Variations:

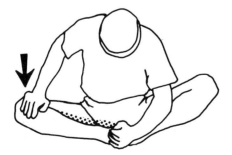

Hold on to your feet with one hand, with your elbow on the inside of the lower leg to hold down and stabilize the leg. Now, with your other hand on the inside of your leg (*not on knee*), gently push your leg downward to isolate and stretch this side of the groin. This is a very good isolation stretch for people who want to limber up a tight groin so that the knees can fall more naturally downward.

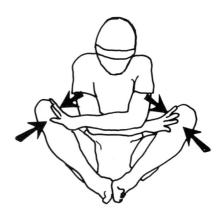

With hands supplying slight resistance on insides of opposite thighs, try to bring knees together, just enough to contract the muscles in the groin. Hold this stabilized tension for 5-8 seconds, then relax and stretch the groin as in the preceding stretches. This will help relax a tight groin area. This technique of tension-relax-stretch is valuable for athletes who have had groin problems.

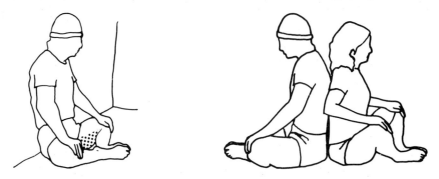

Another way to stretch the tight muscles of the groin area is to sit against a wall or couch: something that will give support. With your back straight and the soles of your feet together, use your hands to push gently down on the inside of your thighs (*not on* the knees, just above them). Push gently until you get a good, even stretch. Hold and relax for 30 seconds.

It is also possible to do this stretch with a partner. Sit back-to-back for stability.

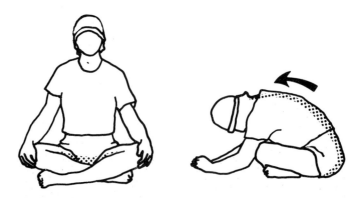

If you've had trouble sitting cross-legged you'll find that these groin stretches will start to make that position easier for you. A good relaxing position that stretches the back and inside of the legs is done by first sitting in the crossed-leg position and then leaning forward until you feel a good comfortable stretch. Get your elbows out in front of you if you can. Hold and relax. This really feels good in the lower back and is a simple stretch for most people.

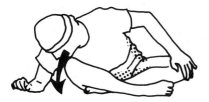

A variation is to move your upper body over your knee instead of straight ahead. This is good for your hips. Think of bending from the hips.

The Spinal Twist:

The spinal twist is good for the upper back, lower back, side of hips, and rib cage. It is also beneficial for internal organs and will help keep your waist-line trim. It will aid in your ability to turn to the side or look behind you without having to turn your entire body.

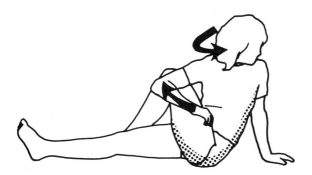

Sit with your right leg straight. Bend your left leg, cross your left foot over and rest it to the outside of your right knee. Then bend your right elbow and rest it on the outside of your upper left thigh, just above the knee. During the stretch use the elbow to keep this leg stationary with controlled pressure to the inside.

Now, with your left hand resting behind you, slowly turn your head to look over your left shoulder, and at the same time rotate your upper body toward your left hand and arm. As you turn your upper body, think of turning your hips in the same direction (though your hips won't move because your right elbow is keeping the left leg stationary). This should give you a stretch in your lower back and side of hip. Hold for 15 seconds. Do both sides. Don't hold your breath; breathe easily.

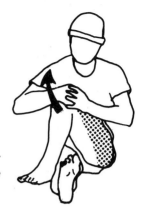

Variation: Pull your knee across your body toward your opposite shoulder until an easy stretch is felt on the side of the hip. Hold for 30 seconds. Do both sides.

People tend to spend more time on the first leg, arm, or area they stretch, and they usually will stretch their "easy" or more flexible side first. Because of this natural tendency more time is spent on the "good" side and less on the "bad" side. To even out the difference in flexibility in your body, stretch your tight side first. This will help you limber up considerably.

SUMMARY

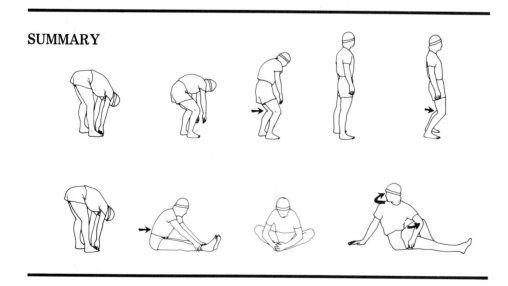

AT THIS TIME LET'S GO OVER SOME OF THE BASIC TECHNIQUES OF STRETCHING:

· Don't stretch too far, especially in the beginning. Get a slight stretch and increase it after you feel yourself relax.
· Hold a stretch in a comfortable position; the stretch tension should subside as you hold it.
· Breathe slowly, deeply and naturally—exhale as you bend forward. Do not stretch to a point where you cannot breathe normally.
· Do not bounce. Bouncing tightens the very muscles you are trying to stretch. Stretch and hold it.
· Think about the area being stretched. Feel the stretch. If the tension becomes greater as you stretch, you are over-stretching. Ease off into a more comfortable position.
· Do not try to be flexible. Just learn to stretch properly and flexibility will come with time. Flexibility is only one of the many by-products of stretching.

OTHER THINGS TO BE AWARE OF:

· We are different every day. Some days we are more tight or loose than other days.
· You have control over what you feel by what you do.
· Regularity and relaxation are the most important factors in stretching. If you start stretching regularly you will naturally become more active and fit.
· Don't compare yourself with others. Even if you are tight or inflexible, don't let this stop you from stretching and improving yourself.
· Proper stretching means stretching within your own limits, relaxed, and without comparisons.
· Stretching keeps your body ready for movement.
· Stretch whenever you feel like it. It will always make you feel good.

STRETCHES FOR THE BACK

It is best to stretch on a firm but not hard surface, especially when doing these stretches for the back. If you are on a surface that is too hard you won't be able to relax as easily.

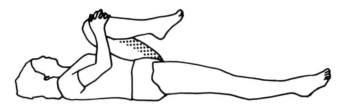

Lie on your back and pull your left leg toward your chest. Keep the back of your head on the mat if possible, but don't strain. If you can't do it with your head down, don't worry. Keep the other leg as straight as possible, without straining. Do this to both sides. This will help to slowly loosen up the back muscles and hamstrings. Hold for 30 seconds.

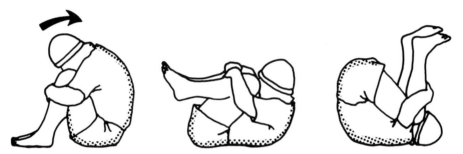

Don't do this on a hard surface, but use a mat or rug. In a sitting position hold your knees with your hands and pull them to your chest. Gently roll up and down your spine, keeping your chin down toward your chest. This will further stretch the muscles along the spine.

Try to roll evenly and with control. Roll back and forth 4-8 times or until you feel your back start to limber up. Do not rush. Do not over-do, but instead, *gradually* develop your physical well-being.

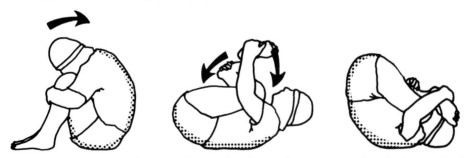

Next is the spinal roll with alternating lower leg cross and pull-down. Begin your roll in the same sitting position as in the previous straight spinal roll. As you roll backwards, cross your lower legs and, at the same time, pull your feet (from the outside) toward your chest. Then, release your feet as you roll up to a sitting position with your feet together and uncrossed. (Always start each roll with the legs uncrossed.) On each repetition, alternate the crossing of your lower legs so that, with the pull-down phase of the roll, the lower back will be stretched evenly on both sides. Do 6-8 repetitions.

Caution: *If your back is extremely tight, do not stretch it too much at the beginning.* Get down the technique and balance; always pull your legs toward your chest with a constant, easy pull. Work slow and easy, concentrating on relaxing and developing patience.

Take your time in stretching your back. Do not rush through the stretches. Concentrate on relaxing in every stretch that you do. Find a stretch that feels good. Do not torture yourself.

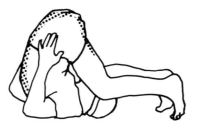

The Legs-overhead Stretch: Now that the back muscles have been stretched and loosened up somewhat, slowly roll back with your feet and legs over your head. Keep your hands on your hips for support and control of the stretch. Try to find a position that is comfortable and allows you to breathe naturally. Do not hold your breath or stretch in a position that cuts off your oxygen supply. Once you find a comfortable position, relax.

A good way to stretch your back is to find a comfortable position, increase the stretch by slightly changing your position, and then return to the original comfortable position. Learn to stretch and relax. Don't be in a hurry.

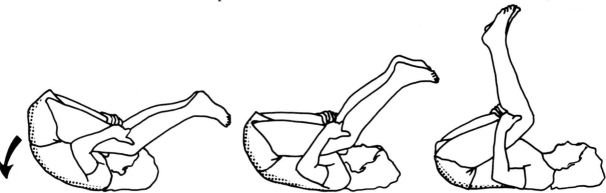

With legs overhead, roll down slowly, trying to roll on each vertebra, one at a time. At first you will probably come down fast, but if you practice, your back will limber up so you will be able to lower yourself slowly, vertebra after vertebra.

Put your hands directly behind your knees and *keep your knees bent* as you roll down. Use your arms and hands to hold your legs still. This will give you greater control of the speed at which you lower yourself. Keep your head on the floor. You may need to move your head slightly for balance.

Rolling out of the legs-overhead position slowly like this is a good way to find out exactly what part of your back is the tightest. The part or parts of your back which are the hardest to lower slowly are the tightest. But you can stretch the tightness and inflexibility out of the spine if you spend a little time working on it gently every day.

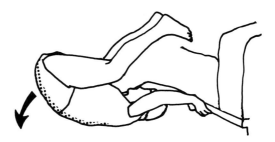

To intensify the stretch in your back when lowering yourself from legs-overhead, place your arms over your head and hold onto something that is stable like the edge of the mat, or a heavy piece of furniture. Now, with a slight bend in your arms and your knees fairly bent, slowly lower yourself one vertebra at a time. By holding onto something with your hands you are able to stretch the back more fully. Go slowly and under control.

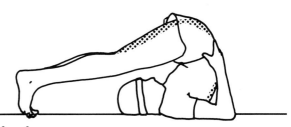

There are many variations of legs-overhead:

If you are unable to touch the floor behind you with your toes, just find a position that is comfortable with your knees bent.

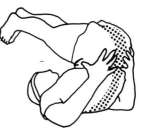

Or bend your knees and spread your legs to rest on either side of your head.

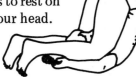

If you are fairly flexible you may do legs-overhead with your legs straight and fingers touching toes. This stretch will help stretch the hamstrings farther and increase the stretch in the middle to lower back.

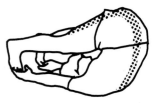

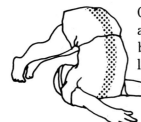

Or you could put your arms in front of your body as you keep your legs almost straight.

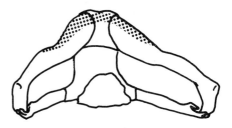

It is also possible to stretch your groin in the legs-overhead position.

If your abdominal muscles are fairly strong, start experimenting with a semi-shoulder stand with hands on hips for balance. Develop balance.

In all of these positions you will be able to feel and see the middle of your body. If these stretches are hard to do, leaving you little room for breathing, you may be carrying too much extra weight in the wrong place. When the body can be relaxed in any of these variations of legs-overhead then it is obviously functioning more efficiently.

Legs-overhead is a good stretch for reducing abdominal fat, stretching the back, and a position for elevating the feet which helps in the re-circulation of blood in the lower limbs.

Many of us get tired in the lower back from hours of standing and sitting. One position which helps to reduce this tension is the squat.

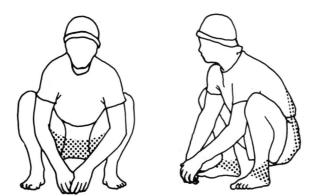

From a standing position, squat down with your feet flat and toes pointed out at approximately 15° angles. Your heels should be 4-12 inches apart, depending on how limber you are, or as you become familiar with stretching, depending on exactly what parts of your body you want to stretch. The squat stretches the front part of the lower legs, the knees, back, ankles, Achilles tendons, and deep groin. Keep knees to the outside of your shoulders. Knees should be directly above big toes in this squat position. Hold comfortably for 30 seconds. For many people this will be easy, for others very difficult.

Variations: At first there may be a problem with balance: usually falling backwards because of tight ankles and tight Achilles tendons. If you are unable to squat as shown on p. 65, there are other ways to learn this position.

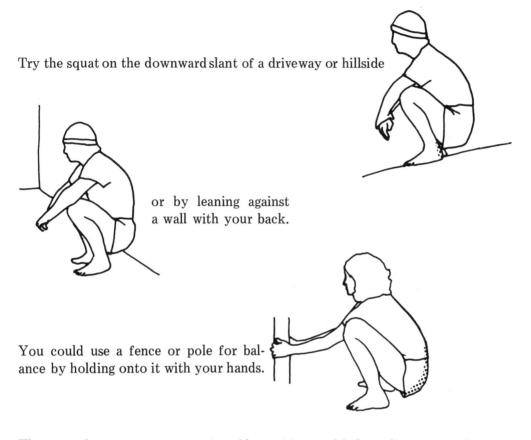

Try the squat on the downward slant of a driveway or hillside

or by leaning against a wall with your back.

You could use a fence or pole for balance by holding onto it with your hands.

The squat becomes a very comfortable position and helps relieve any tightness in the lower back.

Be careful if you have had any knee problems. If pain is present discontinue this stretch.

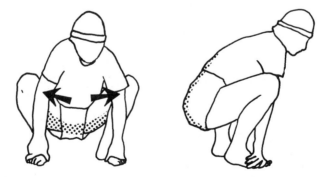

To increase the stretch in the groin, place your elbows on the inside of your upper legs, gently push outward with both elbows as you bend slightly forward from your hips. Your thumbs should be on the inside of your feet with your fingers along the outside borders of the feet. Hold stretch for 20 seconds. Do not overstretch. If you have trouble balancing, elevate your heels slightly.

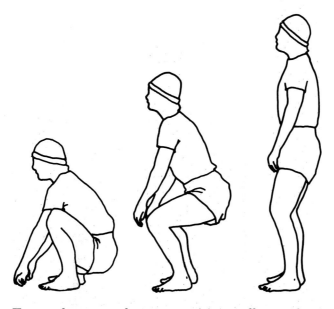

To stand up from the squat position, pull your chin in slightly and raise straight up *with your quadriceps doing all the work and back straight*. Do not dip your head forward as you stand up: this puts too much pressure on your lower back.

SUMMARY

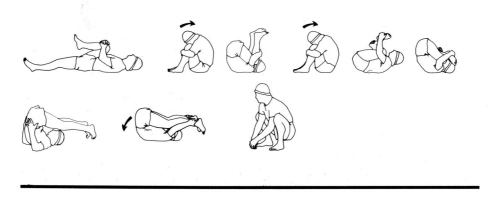

Holding the right stretch tensions for a period of time allows the body to adapt to these new positions. Soon the area being stretched will adapt to the slight tension and gradually the the body can and will assume the new positions without the tightness formerly felt.

ELEVATING YOUR FEET

Elevation of the feet before and after activity is a great way to revitalize your legs. It helps keep the legs light with plenty of consistent energy for everyday living and activity. It is a wonderful way to rest and relax tired, stood-on feet. It helps the entire body feel good. And it is a simple way to help prevent or relieve varicose veins. I recommend elevating the feet at least twice a day for at least 2-3 minutes for revitalization and relaxation.

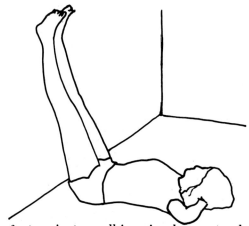

Lying on the floor and resting your feet against a wall is a simple way to elevate your feet. Keep your lower back flat. Your butt should be at least 3 inches from the wall.

If there isn't a wall close by you can elevate the feet from the legs-overhead position.

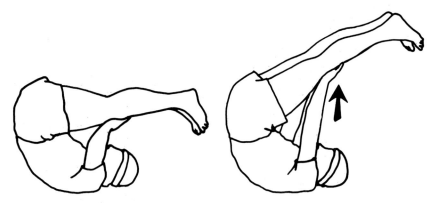

Put the palms of your hands on your knees with fingers pointed toward your toes. Lock or straighten out your arms. If you relax at the hips, your arms will take care of the weight of your legs. This is a very relaxing position. In Hatha yoga it is called the "pose of tranquility." There is a balancing point at the back of your head and the top of the spine when you are in this position. The balance is difficult to find but it is not as hard as it might seem at first. Give it at least 10-12 good tries. A little practice makes it simple.

Shoulder stands are also excellent for elevating the feet. When you start working on shoulder stands it is important to have strong abdominal muscles.

Keep your hands on the back of your hips and try to keep your legs over your head. Your hands on your hips will give you balance and support. Tighten your gluteus muscles for support of the pelvic area and for a more upright posture.

After this position becomes easier and your abdominals become stronger, you can release your arms and either place them over your head, behind your back, or straight along your legs. This last position is an advanced and more difficult position.

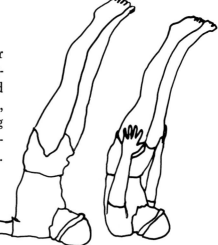

Begin doing shoulder stands for only a few seconds. Gradually increase the time that you hold your feet above your head.

We may know that stretching and regular exercising are beneficial, but knowledge alone is not enough. *Doing* is what is important, for what good is knowledge if we do not use it to live more fully?

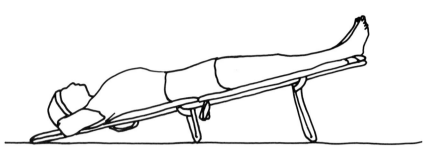

A great way to elevate your feet is to lie on a slant board (available through Sears Roebuck catalog). Don't do any exercises on the slant board, just lie there and relax for about 5 minutes, gradually increasing the time to 15-20 minutes.

This is a good position for pulling in your stomach and being thin. The internal organs will gradually fall back into a normal position. For people who want to look and feel thin, the slant board is excellent.

When getting up from the slant board, sit up for 2-3 minutes before you stand. You should get up slowly from all positions with feet elevated so you don't become dizzy.

Variations:

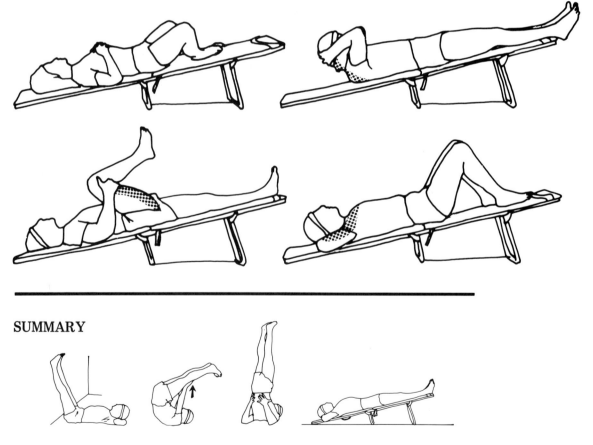

SUMMARY

STANDING STRETCHES FOR LEGS AND HIPS

This series of stretches will help your walking and running. It will give flexibility and energy to the legs. All of the stretches can be done standing up.

To stretch your calf, stand a little ways from a solid support and lean on it with your forearms, head resting on hands. Bend one leg and place your foot on the ground in front of you, with the other leg straight behind. Slowly move your hips forward, keeping your lower back flat. Be sure to keep the heel of the straight leg on the ground, with toes pointed straight ahead or slightly turned in as you hold the stretch. Hold an easy stretch for 30 seconds. Do not bounce. Stretch other leg.

To create a stretch for the calf and Achilles tendon, lower your hips downward as you slightly bend your knee. Be sure to keep your back flat. Your back foot should be slightly toed-in or straight ahead during the stretch. Keep your heel down. This stretch is good for developing ankle flexibility. Hold stretch 25 seconds. The Achilles tendon area needs only a *slight feeling of stretch*.

To stretch the outside of the hip, start from the same position as in the calf stretch. Stretch the right side of your hip by slightly turning your right hip to the inside. Project the side of your right hip to the side as you lean your shoulders very slightly in the opposite direction of your hips. Hold an even stretch for 25 seconds. Do both sides. Keep foot of back leg pointed straight ahead with heel flat on ground.

The Achilles tendon and ankle may be stretched several ways. I have already discussed using a wall for support and the Achilles tendon stretch from the toe pointer position (see p. 47). If you want to stretch this area further you can use a curb or the stairs.

Place the ball of your foot on the edge of a curb or stair, with the rest of the foot hanging down over the edge. Lower the heel below the level of the stair or curb. Go slowly and work on balance. You may need to hold on to the stair railing or a car for balance. The leg of the Achilles tendon and ankle being stretched should be kept straight. Stretch in the easy phase only. Hold for 20 seconds.

Also do the stretch with your knee slightly bent to change the stretch feeling to a higher part of the Achilles tendon.

This is a good stretch to do after a hard workout or when the calves and Achilles tendons feel extremely tight. It can be done practically anywhere and adds some life to the lower legs.

Hold on to something and pull your knee toward your chest. Do not lean forward at the waist or hips. This gently stretches your upper hamstrings, butt, and hips. The foot on the ground should be pointed straight ahead with the knee slightly bent (1 inch). Hold an easy stretch for 30 seconds. Do both legs.

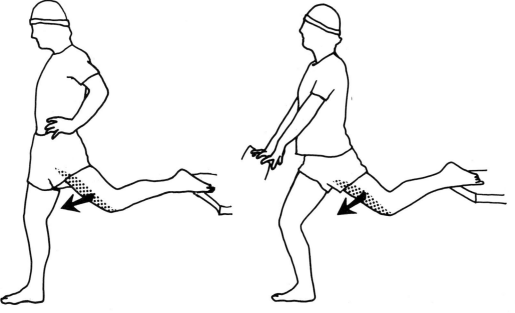

Place the ball of your foot up on a secure support of some kind (wall, fence, table). Keep the down leg pointed straight ahead. Now bend the knee of the up leg as you move your hips forward. This should stretch your groin, hamstrings, and front of hip. Hold for 30 seconds. Do both sides. If possible, for balance and control, use your hands to hold on to the support. This stretch will make it easier to lift your knees.

Variation: Instead of having the foot on the ground pointed straight ahead, turn it to the side (parallel to the support), then stretch as above. This stretches the inside of the upper legs. Hold for 25 seconds.

Extend your foot in back of you, setting the top of it on a table, fence or bar behind you at a comfortable height. Think of pulling your leg through (moving your leg forward) from the front of your hip to create a stretch for the front of the hip (*iliopsoas*) and quadriceps. Flex your butt (*gluteus*) muscles as you do this stretch. Keep the down knee slightly bent (1 inch) and upper body vertical. The foot on the ground should be pointed straight ahead. You can change the stretch by slightly bending the knee of the supporting leg a little more. Hold an easy stretch for 20 seconds. Learn to feel balanced and comfortable in this stretch through relaxed practice.

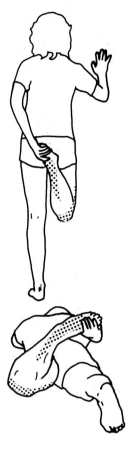

To stretch the quad and knee, hold the top of your *right* foot with your *left* hand and gently pull your heel toward your buttocks. The knee bends at a natural angle when you hold your foot with the opposite hand. This is good to use in knee rehabilitation and with problem knees. Hold for 30 seconds, each leg.

A variation of this stretch can be done lying on your stomach. Be sure to stretch without pain. Reach behind you with your hand and hold the top of your opposite foot between the ankle joint and toes. Gently pull your heel toward the middle of your buttocks. Hold 8-12 seconds.

Remember to stretch under control. Start in a place that is fairly easy and go from there. Improvement and results will occur faster if you go from an easy stretch to a developmental stretch. Let yourself limber up slowly. Remember, straining will keep you from fully realizing the many benefits of stretching.

Place the back of your heel on a tree, fence, table, or large rock which is about waist high or at a comfortable height. You want to keep the leg that is raised straight, so don't use something that is too high. If you are at a track, a hurdle works well because it is usually adjustable in height. The leg on the ground should be slightly bent at the knee (1 inch), with your foot pointed forward as in a proper running or walking position.

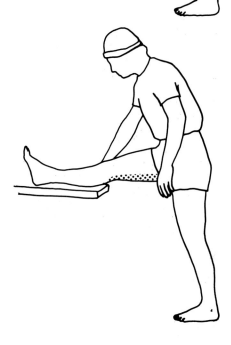

Now, while looking straight ahead, slowly bend forward at the waist until you feel a good stretch in the back of the raised leg. Hold and relax. Find the easy stretch, relax, and then increase it. This is very good for running or walking.

Variation: If you cannot easily touch your toes, rest more of your leg up on a table or platform of some kind that is at a comfortable height for you. Then you will be able to use the side of the table or ledge for balance and support as you get the right feeling of stretch in the hamstrings.

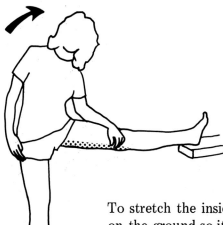

To stretch the inside of your raised leg, turn the foot that is on the ground so it is parallel to the support. Face your upper body in the same direction as your down foot and turn your left hip slightly to the inside. Slowly bend sideways with your left shoulder going toward your left knee. This should stretch the inside of your upper leg. Hold an easy stretch for 15 seconds and a developmental stretch for 20 seconds. Be sure to keep the knee of the down leg slightly bent. Do both legs.

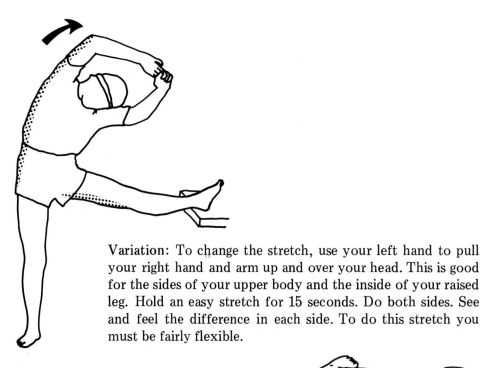

Variation: To change the stretch, use your left hand to pull your right hand and arm up and over your head. This is good for the sides of your upper body and the inside of your raised leg. Hold an easy stretch for 15 seconds. Do both sides. See and feel the difference in each side. To do this stretch you must be fairly flexible.

To change the stretch, bend at the waist toward the foot on the ground. The raised leg should remain straight but will turn to the inside as you bend over. Hold this position and stretch the hamstrings of the supporting leg. The knee of that leg should be slightly bent (1 inch) during the stretch. Hold an easy stretch for 20 seconds.

If you want to stretch the groin area of the raised leg, bend the knee of the supporting leg and keep the raised leg straight. If you can, rest your hands on the ground to give you added balance. Hold an easy stretch for 20 seconds.

SUMMARY

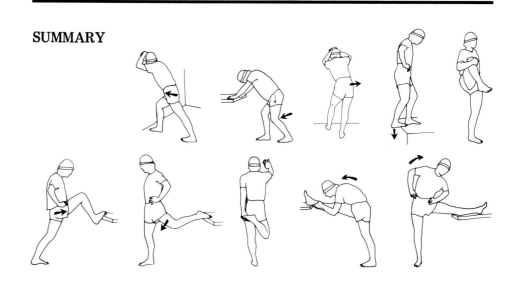

It is important to maintain good flexibility throughout our lives, so that as we get older we can avoid the problems that go with stiff joints, tight muscles and bad posture. One of the striking characteristics of aging is the loss of range of motion, and stretching is perhaps the single most important thing you can do to keep your body limber.

STANDING STRETCHES FOR THE UPPER BODY

These next stretches are excellent for trimming the waistline. They will stretch the muscles along your side from your arm to your hips. They are done standing up, and you can do them any time, and anywhere.

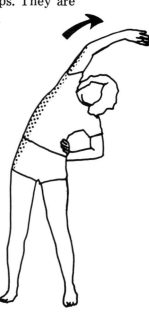

Stand with your feet about shoulder-width apart and toes pointed straight ahead. Keeping your knees slightly bent (1 inch), place one hand on your hip for support while you extend your other arm up and over your head. Now slowly bend at your waist to the side, toward the hand on your hip. Move slowly; feel a good stretch. Hold and relax. Gradually increase the amount of time you are able to hold the stretch (easy stretch for 10-15 seconds). Always come out of a stretch slowly and under control. No quick or jerky movements.

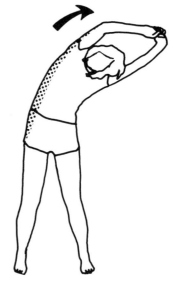

Instead of using your hand on your hip for support, extend both arms overhead. Grasp your right hand with your left hand and bend slowly to the left, using your left arm to gently pull the right arm over the head and down toward the ground.

By using one arm to pull the other you can increase the stretch along your sides and along the spine. *Do not overstretch.* Hold an easy stretch for 8-10 seconds.

This stretch for the upper body stretches the muscles laterally along the spine.

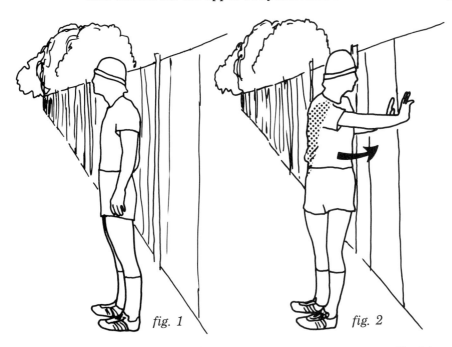

fig. 1   fig. 2

Stand about 12-24 inches away from a fence or wall with your back towards it (fig. 1). With your feet about shoulder-width apart and toes pointed straight ahead, slowly turn your upper body around until you can easily place your hands on the fence or wall at about shoulder height (fig. 2). Turn in one direction and touch the wall, return to the starting position, and then turn in the opposite direction and touch the wall. Do not force yourself to turn any farther than is fairly comfortable. If you have a knee problem, do this stretch very slowly and cautiously. Be relaxed and do not force. Hold for 10-20 seconds. Gradually increase the length of time you hold this stretch. Keep knees slightly bent (1 inch).

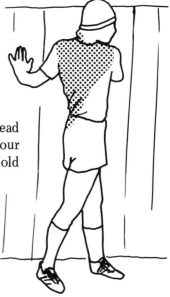

Variation: To change the stretch, turn your head and look over your right shoulder. Try to keep your hips facing forward and parallel to the fence. Hold an easy stretch for 10 seconds. Do both sides.

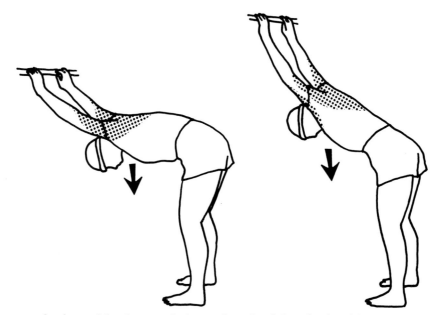

Another good upper body and back stretch is to place both hands shoulder-width apart on a fence or ledge and let your upper body drop down as you keep your knees slightly bent (1 inch). (Always bend your knees when coming out of this stretch.) Your hips should be directly above your feet.

Now, bend your knees just a bit more and feel the stretch change. Place your hands at different heights and change the area of the stretch. After you become familiar with this stretch it is possible to really stretch the spine. Great to do if you have been slumping in the upper back and shoulders all day. This will take some of the kinks out of a tired upper back. Find a stretch that you can hold for at least 30 seconds.

The top of the refrigerator or a file cabinet are good to use for this stretch. Do it slowly. It can be done practically anywhere: all it takes is a little thought and some doing.

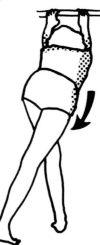

To increase and change the area of the stretch in another way, bring one leg behind and across the midline of your body as you lean in the opposite direction. This will stretch those hard-to-reach areas of the upper body.

I find these arm and shoulder stretches to be very good before and after running. They allow for a relaxed upper body and a freer arm swing. They are also good to do during weight-lifting workouts or as a warm-up for any upper body activity such as tennis, baseball, handball, etc.

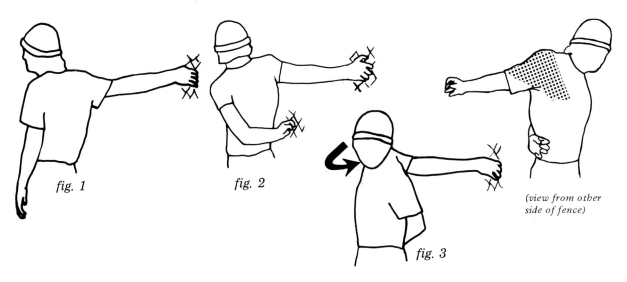

fig. 1

fig. 2

fig. 3

(view from other side of fence)

This stretch is for the front of the shoulders and arms. You need a chain-linked fence, doorway, or wall. Face the fence and hold onto it (or press against it) with your right hand at shoulder level (fig. 1). Next, bring your other arm around your back and grab the fence (or whatever you are using) as in fig. 2. Now, look over your left shoulder in the direction of your right hand. Keep your shoulder close to the fence as you slowly turn your head (fig. 3). Trying to look at your right hand behind you gives you a stretch in the front of the shoulders.

Stretch the other side. Do it slowly and under control. The feeling of a good stretch is what is important: *not how far you can stretch.*

Variation: From the previous position, stretch your arm and shoulder at various angles. Each angle will stretch the arm and shoulder differently. Hold for 10 seconds.

Here is another stretch you can do while using a chain-linked fence or wall for support and balance.

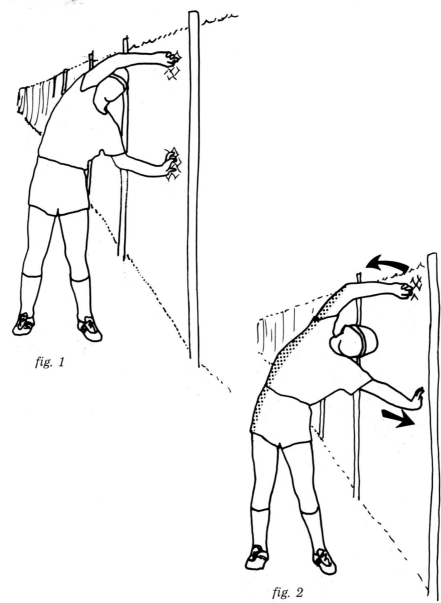

fig. 1

fig. 2

Hold on to the fence about waist-high with your left hand. Now reach over your head with your right arm and grab the fence with your right hand. Your left arm will be slightly bent with the right arm extended (fig. 1). Keep knees slightly bent (1 inch).

To stretch your waistline and sides, straighten your left arm and pull over with your (upper) right arm (fig. 2). Hold for 10 seconds. Do both sides.

Slowly go into each stretch and slowly come out of each stretch. Do not bob, jerk, or bounce. Keep your stretching fluid and under control.

SUMMARY

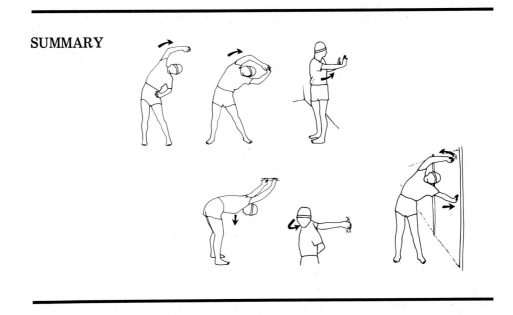

Enjoy stretching by the way it feels. If you torture yourself with drastic tensions because you think you should be flexible, you deprive yourself of the true benefits of stretching. If you stretch correctly, you'll find the more you stretch, the easier it becomes, and the easier you stretch, the more you will naturally enjoy it.

STRETCHING ON A CHIN BAR

With the help of gravity, it is possible to get a fine stretch on a chin bar.

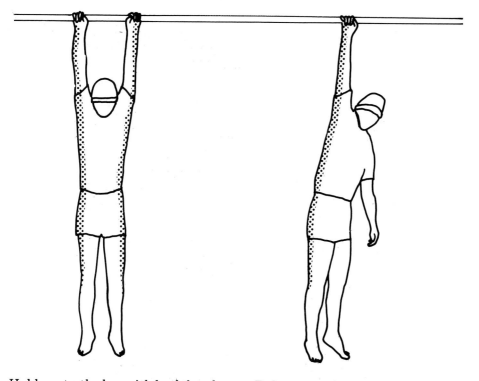

Hold on to the bar with both hands, relax your chin forward as you hang with feet off the ground. A great stretch for the back. Begin holding for 10 seconds, gradually increasing to at least 60 seconds. A strong grip will make this stretch easier.

Release one hand and hang by only one hand. This will stretch the shoulder, ribs, and side of upper back. Hold and relax. Again, be gradual in your approach. Begin holding this stretch for 5 seconds. Do not hang too long at the beginning. This is a good stretch if you let yourself relax.

Caution: *Do not attempt this stretch if you have or have had an injury in the shoulder area.*

STRETCHES FOR THE UPPER BODY USING A TOWEL

Most of us have a towel in our hands at least once a day. A towel can aid in stretching the arms, shoulders, and chest.

Grab the towel near both ends so that you can move it, with straight arms, up and over your head and down behind your back. Do not strain or force it. Your hands should be far enough apart to allow for relatively free movement up and over your head and down behind your back.

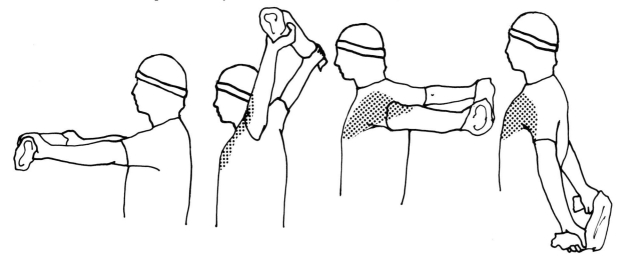

To increase the stretch, move your hands slightly closer together and, keeping the arms straight, repeat the movement. Go slowly and feel the stretch. Do not overstretch. If you are unable to go through the full movement of up, over, and behind while keeping your arms straight, then your hands are too close together. Move them farther apart.

You can hold the stretch at any place during this movement. This will isolate and add further stretch to the muscles of that particular area. For example: if your chest is tight and sore, it is possible to isolate the stretch there by holding the towel at shoulder level with arms straight behind you, as shown above. Hold for 10-20 seconds.

Stretching is not a contest. You needn't compare yourself with others, because we are all different. Moreover, each day we are different: some days we are more limber than others. Stretch comfortably, within *your* limits, and you will begin to feel the flow of energy that comes from proper stretching.

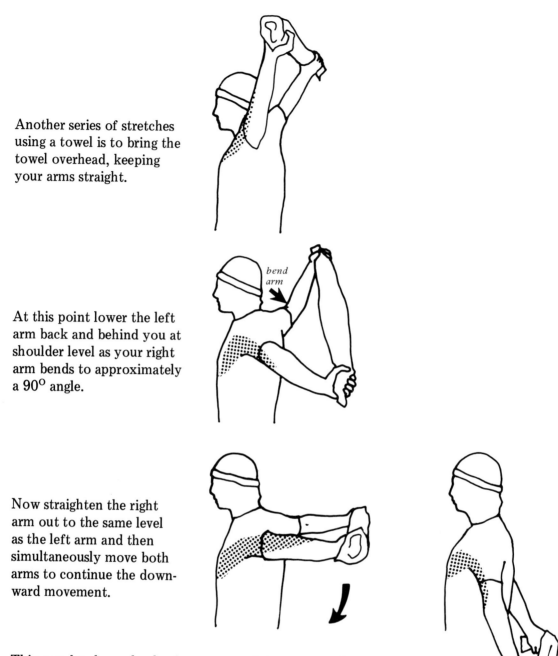

Another series of stretches using a towel is to bring the towel overhead, keeping your arms straight.

At this point lower the left arm back and behind you at shoulder level as your right arm bends to approximately a 90° angle.

bend arm

Now straighten the right arm out to the same level as the left arm and then simultaneously move both arms to continue the downward movement.

This can be done slowly, in one complete movement, or you can stop at any point to increase the stretch in that particular area. Do this complete movement toward the other side by lowering your right arm first.

As you become more flexible you will be able to hold the towel with your hands closer together. But again, do not strain.

I think that limberness in the shoulders and arms really helps tennis, running, walking, and of course swimming (to name only a few activities where you need this flexibility). Stretching the chest area reduces muscle tension and tightness and increases circulation. It is actually very simple to stretch and keep the upper body limber, if you do it *regularly*.

SITTING STRETCHES

Here is a series of stretches you can do while sitting. They are good for people who work at office jobs. You can relieve tension and energize parts of your body that have become stiff from sitting.

Interlace your fingers, then straighten your arms out in front of you with palms facing out. Feel the stretch in arms and through upper part of back (shoulder blades). Hold stretch for 20 seconds. Do at least twice.

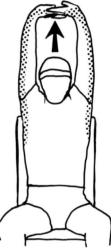

Interlace fingers, then turn palms upward above your head as you straighten your arms. Think of elongating your arms as you feel a stretch through your arms and upper sides of rib cage. Hold only a stretch that feels good. Do three times. Hold for 10 seconds.

With arms extended overhead, hold on to the outside of your left hand with right hand and pull your left arm to the side. Keep arms as straight as comfortably possible. This will stretch the arm and side of body and shoulder. Hold for 15 seconds. Do both sides.

Hold your right elbow with your left hand, then gently pull elbow behind head until an easy tension-stretch is felt in shoulder or back of upper arm (*triceps*). Hold an easy stretch for 30 seconds. Do not overstretch.

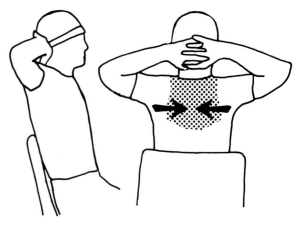

With your fingers interlaced behind your head, keep elbows straight out to side with your upper body in a good, aligned position. Now think of pulling your shoulder blades together to create a feeling of tension through upper back and shoulder blades. Hold feeling of releasing tension for 8-10 seconds, then relax. Do several times. This is good to do when shoulders and upper back are tense or tight.

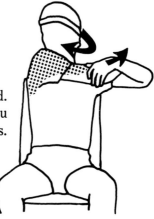

Hold your right arm just above the elbow with your left hand. Now gently pull your elbow toward your left shoulder as you look over your right shoulder. Hold stretch for 10 seconds. Do both sides.

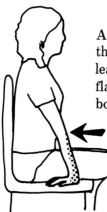

A Stretch for the Forearm: With the palm of your hand flat, thumb to the outside and fingers pointed backward, slowly lean arm back to stretch your forearm. Be sure to keep palms flat. Hold for 35-40 seconds. Do both sides. You can stretch both forearms at the same time, if you wish.

Sitting Stretches for Ankles,
Side of Hip, and Lower Back:

Rotate your ankles while sitting, clockwise and then counter-clockwise. Do one ankle at a time, 20-30 revolutions.

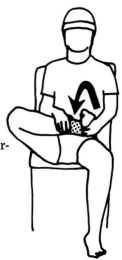

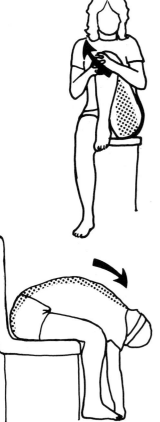

Hold on to your lower left leg just below the knee. Gently pull it toward your chest. To isolate a stretch in the side of your upper leg, use the left arm to pull the bent leg across and toward the opposite shoulder. Hold for 30 seconds at an easy stretch tension. Do both sides.

Lean forward to stretch and to take the pressure off your lower back. Even if you do not feel a stretch, it is still good for circulation. Hold for 45-50 seconds. Put your hands on your thighs to help push your body to an upright position.

Stretches for the Face and Neck:

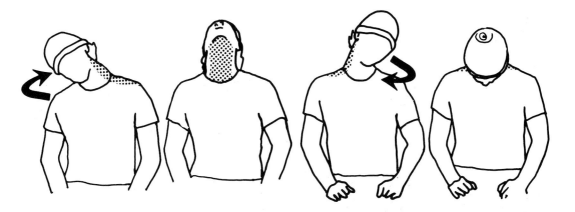

Sit in a position that is comfortable. *Very slowly* roll your head around in a full circle as you keep your back straight. While you are rolling your head around slowly you may feel that you should stop and hold a stretch at a particular place that feels tight. Do so, but don't strain. If you are holding a position, be relaxed and the area will gradually loosen up.

These stretches for your neck will help you sit or stand with better posture when you find you are slouching. See page 183 on sitting.

This stretch may cause people around you to think you are very strange, indeed, but you often find a lot of tension in your face from frowning or squinting because of eye strain.

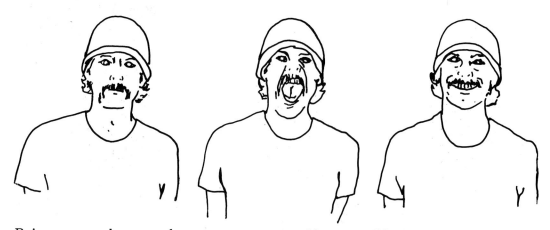

Raise your eyebrows and open your eyes as wide as possible. At the same time, open your mouth to stretch the muscles around your nose and chin and stick your tongue out. Hold this stretch 5-10 seconds. Getting the tension out of the muscles in your face will make you smile.

SUMMARY

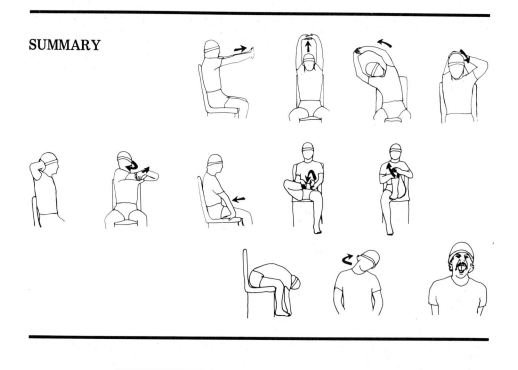

If you don't have much uninterrupted time available, use short periods of stretching (five minutes) every three or four hours. This will help you to feel consistently good throughout the day.

LEG AND GROIN STRETCHES WITH FEET ELEVATED

A wall is very useful for stretching the legs, while you relax on your back. When doing these stretches you must be aware of the easy stretch, then the gradual increase into the developmental stretch. These stretches are easy to do and should be approached this way.

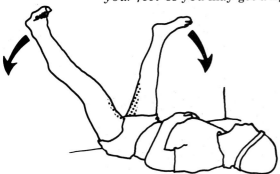

Start with your legs elevated and close together, with your butt about 3-5 inches away from the wall so that your lower back is flat and not arched or off the floor. At first elevate your feet this way for only about one minute. Gradually increase the time until you can do it for 5-8 minutes. If your feet start to go to sleep, roll over on your side and then sit up. (See p. 19 for the proper way to sit up from this position.) *Don't get up quickly after elevating your feet* or you may get a light-headed feeling.

It is possible to stretch your groin from this position by slowly separating your legs, with your heels resting on the wall, until you feel an easy stretch. Hold the stretch 30 seconds and relax.

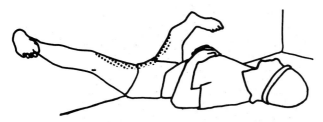

As this position becomes easier with time and patience you can gradually stretch further by lowering your legs. An advanced position is shown here. Do not try to copy this, but stretch within *your* limits. Do not strain. The wall makes it possible to hold these stretches longer in a relaxed, stable position, without wasting energy due to lack of balance.

Remember to keep your butt 3-5 inches from the wall. If you are too close to the wall you may feel tightness in your lower back.

Variation:

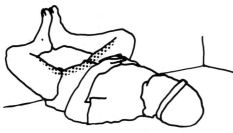

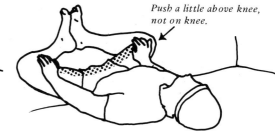

Push a little above knee, not on knee.

Put the soles of your feet together, resting them against the wall. Relax.

To increase the stretch, use your hands to gently push down on the inside of your thighs until you feel a good, easy stretch. Relax while you stretch.

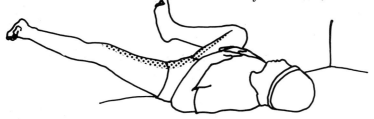

To isolate and increase the stretch in each side of the groin area, straighten one leg out.

To stretch your neck from this position, interlace your fingers behind your head (at about ear level) and gently pull your head forward until you feel an easy stretch. Hold for 5 seconds. Repeat 2 or 3 times. (See p. 25 for further information on neck stretches.)

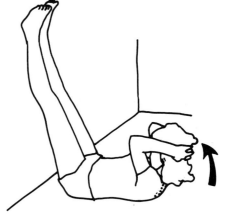

SUMMARY

STRETCHING THE GROIN AND HIPS WITH LEGS APART

The following stretches will make lateral movement easier, help maintain flexibility, and can prevent injuries. Gradually become accustomed to these stretches, which are primarily for the center of your body.

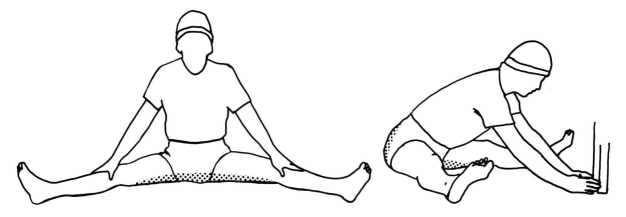

Sit with your feet a comfortable distance apart. To stretch the inside of your upper legs and hips, slowly lean forward from your hips. Be sure to keep your quadriceps relaxed and feet upright. Hold for 35 seconds. Keep your hands out in front of you for balance and stability or hold on to something for greater control.

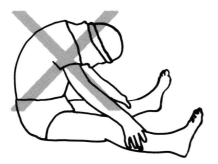

Do not lean forward with your head and shoulders. This will cause your hips to move backward and put pressure on your lower back. If, when you lean forward, you lower back is rounded, it is because your hips, lower back, hamstrings and groin are tight. To bend from your hips correctly, you must keep your back straight.

Don't stretch to be flexible. Stretch to feel good.

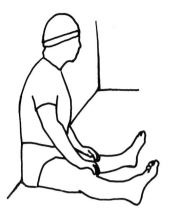
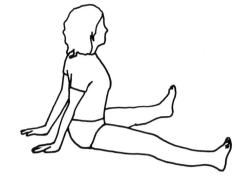

A good way to gradually adapt your hips and lower back to a proper, upright position is to sit with your lower back flat against a wall. Hold an easy stretch for 30 seconds.

Another way is to sit with your hands behind you. Using your arms as a support will help lengthen your spine as you concentrate on moving your hips slightly forward. Hold for 20 seconds.

Do not bend forward until you are able to feel comfortable doing the above. Get your body used to this position before you try to stretch any further.

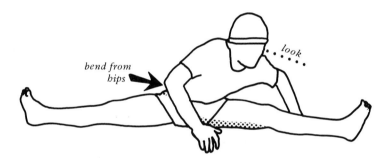

Variation: To stretch your left hamstrings and the right side of your back, slowly bend forward from the hips, toward the foot of your left leg. Keep your chin in and back straight. Hold a good stretch for at least 30-40 seconds. If necessary use a towel.

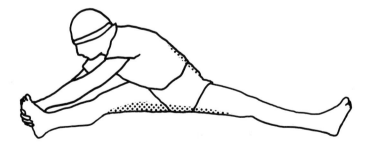

Another variation is to reach across your body with the left hand to the right foot, putting your right hand out to the right side for balance. This will increase the stretch in your hamstrings and in your back, as far up as the shoulder blades and as far down as the hips. Do this across-the-body stretch in both directions.

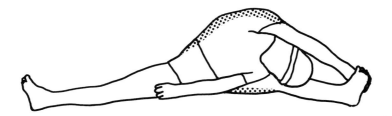

An Advanced Stretch: Reach overhead with hand and grasp opposite foot. Keep your other arm resting close to your body in front of you. This is a good lateral stretch for the back and good for legs. Hold for 30 seconds. Do both sides. Do not overstretch.

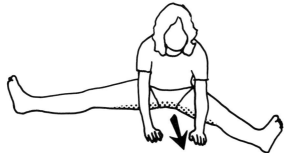

Learn to hold stretch tensions at various angles. Stretch forward, left, and right, then teach yourself to hold stretches at angles toward left center and right center. Use the same leg and upper body alignment as previously described. Hold for 30 seconds. Stretch with complete self-control.

If you feel and look tight doing these stretches do not be discouraged. Stretch without worrying about flexibility. Then you can gradually adapt your body to these new angles with stretch tensions that feel right.

An additional way to stretch the groin:

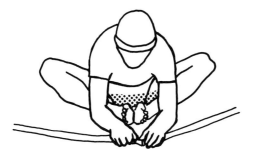

With the soles of your feet together, lean forward and hold on to something near the floor in front of you (this may be the edge of the mat, or the leg of a piece of furniture). Use this object to help you hold a comfortable stretch and to pull yourself forward to increase the stretch. Do not overstretch. Hold and relax for 20-30 seconds. This is a more advanced stretch for the groin.

Holding on to the corner of a gymnastics mat will stabilize your legs and make it easier to hold a stretch when you are sitting with legs apart.

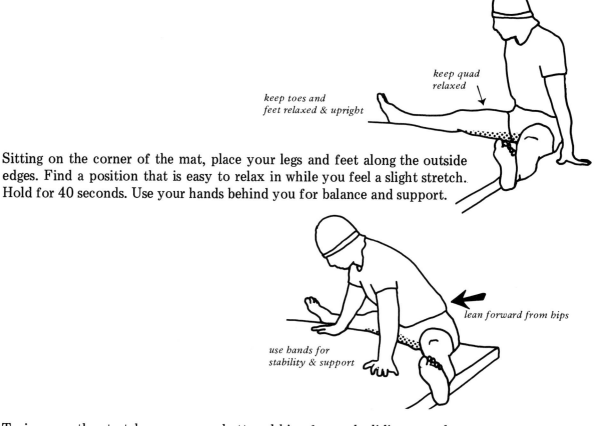

keep quad relaxed

keep toes and feet relaxed & upright

Sitting on the corner of the mat, place your legs and feet along the outside edges. Find a position that is easy to relax in while you feel a slight stretch. Hold for 40 seconds. Use your hands behind you for balance and support.

lean forward from hips

use hands for stability & support

To increase the stretch, move your butt and hips forward, sliding your legs down along the sides of the mat. Keep toes and feet upright. Do not let your legs turn in or out. A good stretch for limbering up groin and hips.

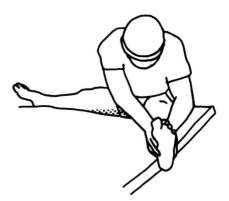

To stretch one leg at a time, sit on the corner of the mat in a comfortable position. Turn to face one foot and bend forward from the hips in that direction. Reach down with your hands and hold some place on your leg which gives you an easy stretch. Think of your chin going toward or just beyond your knee, even though it may not. Relax. Sit up and stretch the other leg in the same way. Stretch your tightest leg first. If necessary, put a towel around the bottom of your foot to help you stretch. Hold an easy stretch 30 seconds. No bouncing. This is good for the hamstrings and lower back.

LEARNING THE SPLITS

This section is for a limited number of people. Unless you are training for gymnastics, dance, or need this extreme flexibility (such as an ice hockey goal-keeper, or a first baseman, or a ballet dancer) the other sections in this book should handle most of your stretching needs. I'm not trying to discourage you, but for everyday living, being able to do the splits is hardly necessary!

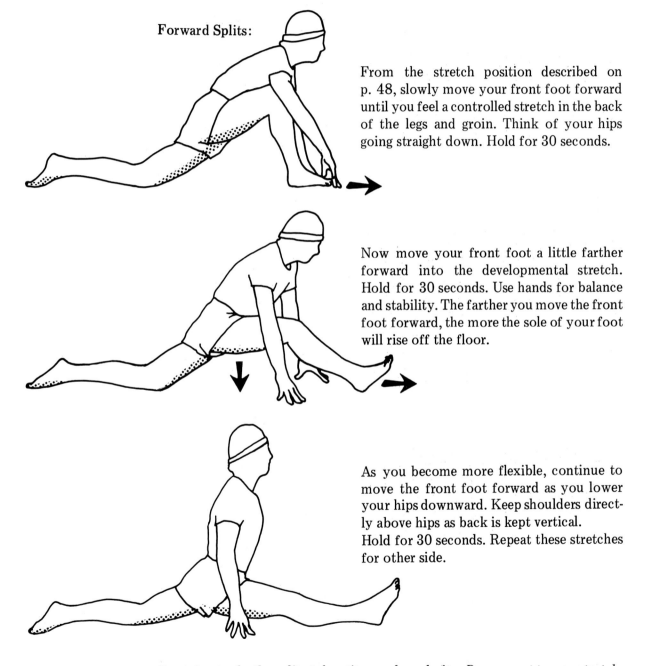

Forward Splits:

From the stretch position described on p. 48, slowly move your front foot forward until you feel a controlled stretch in the back of the legs and groin. Think of your hips going straight down. Hold for 30 seconds.

Now move your front foot a little farther forward into the developmental stretch. Hold for 30 seconds. Use hands for balance and stability. The farther you move the front foot forward, the more the sole of your foot will rise off the floor.

As you become more flexible, continue to move the front foot forward as you lower your hips downward. Keep shoulders directly above hips as back is kept vertical.
Hold for 30 seconds. Repeat these stretches for other side.

Learning to do the splits takes time and regularity. Be sure not to overstretch. Let your body gradually adapt to the changes needed to comfortably accomplish the splits. Do not be in a rush at the expense of injury.

Side Splits:

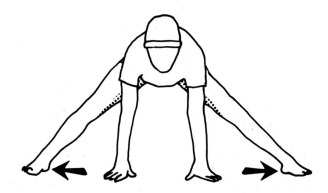

From a standing position with feet pointed straight ahead, gradually spread legs until you feel a stretch on the inside of your upper legs. Think of your hips going straight down. Use hands for balance. Hold an easy stretch for at least 30 seconds.

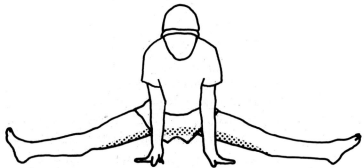

As you become more limber, keep moving your feet apart until the desired stretch is created. As you get lower in this stretch, keep your feet upright, with your heels on the floor: this will keep the stretch feeling on the inside of the upper legs and the extreme tension off the ligaments of the knee. (If you keep your feet flat on the floor there is a possibility of overstretching the inside ligament of the knees.) Hold for 30 seconds. As your body gradually adapts, slowly increase the stretch by lowering your hips down a bit further. *Be careful of overstretching.*

Doing the stretches on p. 91 and p. 96 will help you in learning the splits.

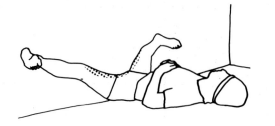

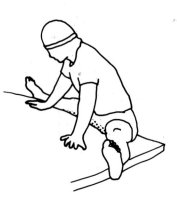

Stretching Routines: Everyday

These stretching routines can be helpful in dealing with the muscular tension and tightness of everyday life. There are ideas about stretching for specific daily activities, such as walking or working, a special routine for those over 50, and stretches to do during spontaneous moments throughout the day. Once you learn how to stretch, you will be able to develop your own routines to suit your own particular needs.

Be sure you are familiar with the individual stretches before you try these routines. For instructions, refer to the page number below each drawing.

In The Morning

Approximately 5 Minutes

Start the day with some relaxed stretches so your body
can function more naturally. Tight and stiff muscles will
feel good from comfortable stretching. It may be helpful
to take a hot shower to get warm before you stretch.

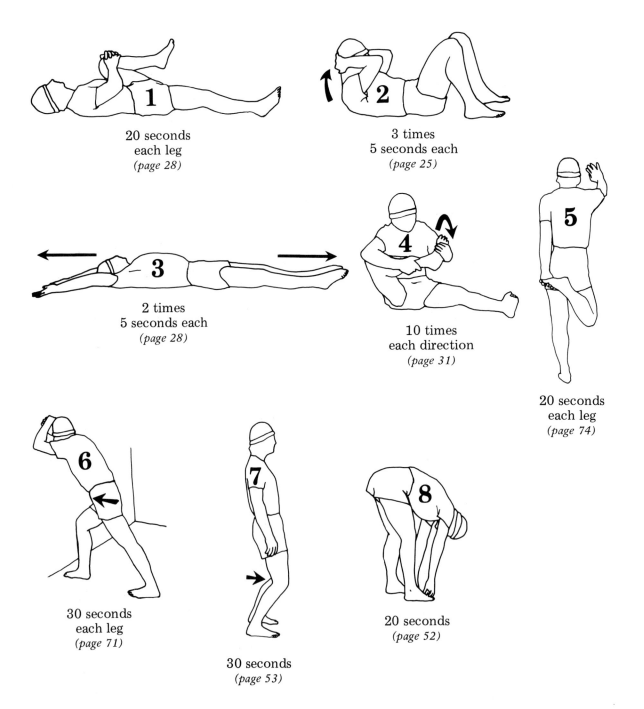

20 seconds
each leg
(page 28)

3 times
5 seconds each
(page 25)

2 times
5 seconds each
(page 28)

10 times
each direction
(page 31)

20 seconds
each leg
(page 74)

30 seconds
each leg
(page 71)

30 seconds
(page 53)

20 seconds
(page 52)

Before and After

Walking

Approximately 7 Minutes

These stretches will make the movements
of walking feel free and easy.

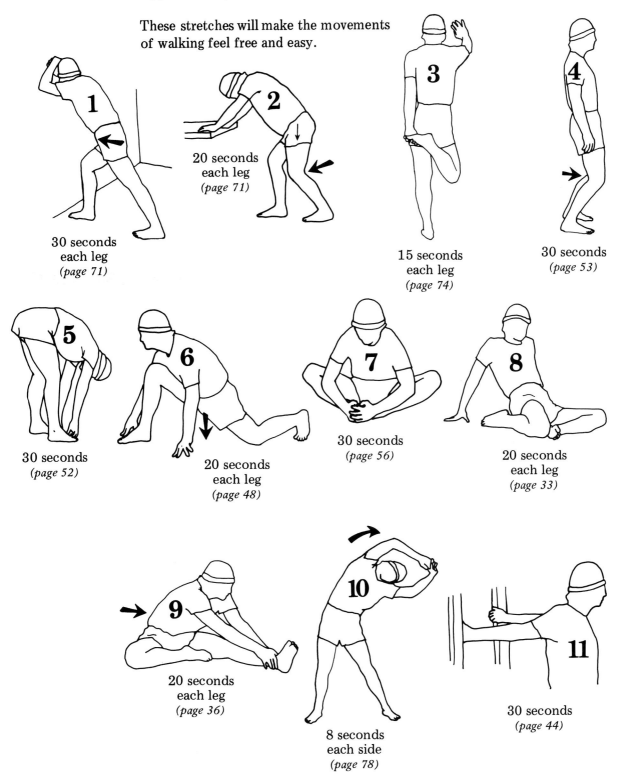

1 30 seconds
each leg
(page 71)

2 20 seconds
each leg
(page 71)

3 15 seconds
each leg
(page 74)

4 30 seconds
(page 53)

5 30 seconds
(page 52)

6 20 seconds
each leg
(page 48)

7 30 seconds
(page 56)

8 20 seconds
each leg
(page 33)

9 20 seconds
each leg
(page 36)

10 8 seconds
each side
(page 78)

11 30 seconds
(page 44)

Everyday Stretches

Approximately 10-15 Minutes

Use these everyday stretches to fine-tune your muscles. This is a general routine that emphasizes stretching and relaxing the muscles most frequently used during the normal day-to-day activities.

In the simple tasks of everyday living, we often use our body in strained or awkward ways, creating stress and tension. A kind of muscular *rigor mortis* sets in. If you can set aside 10-15 minutes every day for stretching, you will offset this accumulated tension so you can use your body with greater ease.

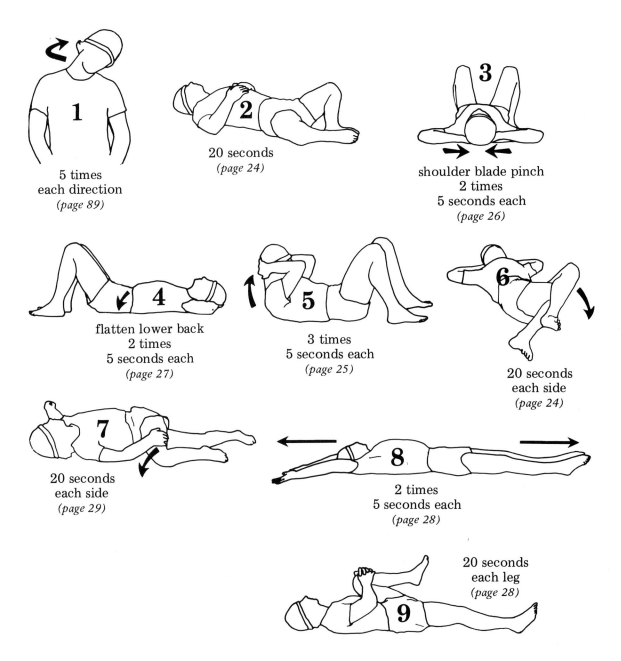

1
5 times
each direction
(page 89)

2
20 seconds
(page 24)

3
shoulder blade pinch
2 times
5 seconds each
(page 26)

4
flatten lower back
2 times
5 seconds each
(page 27)

5
3 times
5 seconds each
(page 25)

6
20 seconds
each side
(page 24)

7
20 seconds
each side
(page 29)

8
2 times
5 seconds each
(page 28)

9
20 seconds
each leg
(page 28)

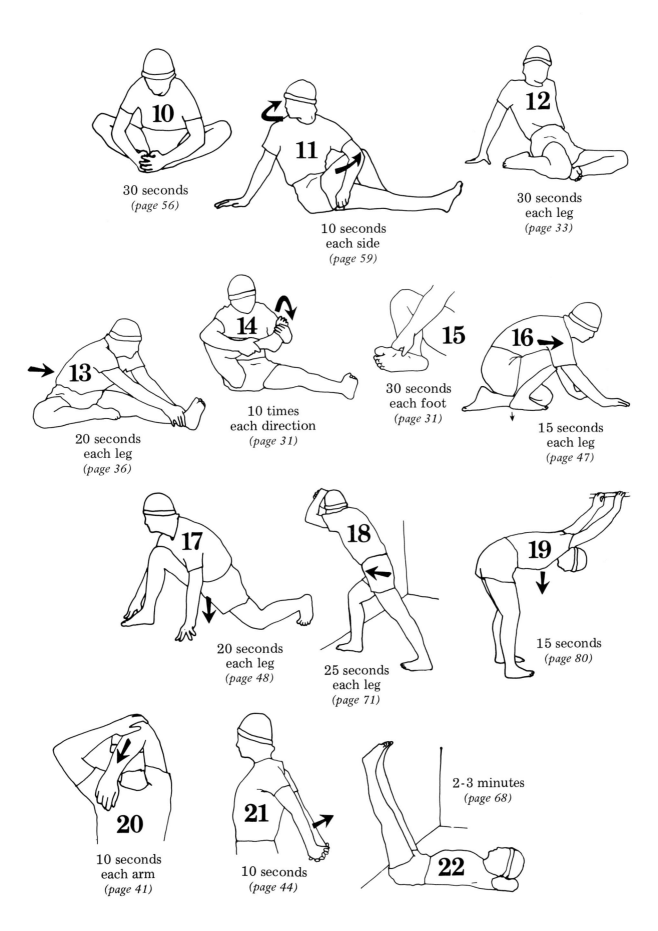

10
30 seconds
(page 56)

11
10 seconds
each side
(page 59)

12
30 seconds
each leg
(page 33)

13
20 seconds
each leg
(page 36)

14
10 times
each direction
(page 31)

15
30 seconds
each foot
(page 31)

16
15 seconds
each leg
(page 47)

17
20 seconds
each leg
(page 48)

18
25 seconds
each leg
(page 71)

19
15 seconds
(page 80)

20
10 seconds
each arm
(page 41)

21
10 seconds
(page 44)

22
2-3 minutes
(page 68)

Stretches For Those

Over 50

Approximately 5-6 Minutes

It is never too late to start stretching. In fact, the older we get, the more important it becomes to stretch on a regular basis.

With age and inactivity, the body gradually loses its range of motion; muscles can lose their elasticity and become weak and tight. But the body has an amazing capacity for the recovery of lost flexibility and strength if a regular program of fitness is followed.

The basic method of stretching is the same regardless of differences in age and flexibility. *Stretching properly means that you do not go beyond your own comfortable limits.* You don't have to try to copy the drawings in this book. Learn to stretch your body without force; stretch by how you feel. It will take time to loosen up tight muscle groups that have been this way for years, but it can be done with patience and regularity. If you have any doubts about what you should be doing, consult your physician *before you start.*

Here is a series of stretches to help restore and maintain flexibility.

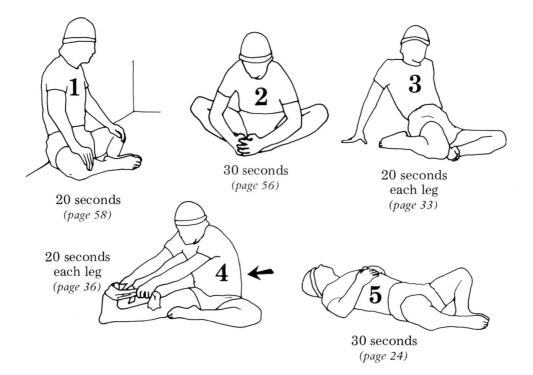

1

20 seconds
(page 58)

2

30 seconds
(page 56)

3

20 seconds
each leg
(page 33)

20 seconds
each leg
(page 36)

4

5

30 seconds
(page 24)

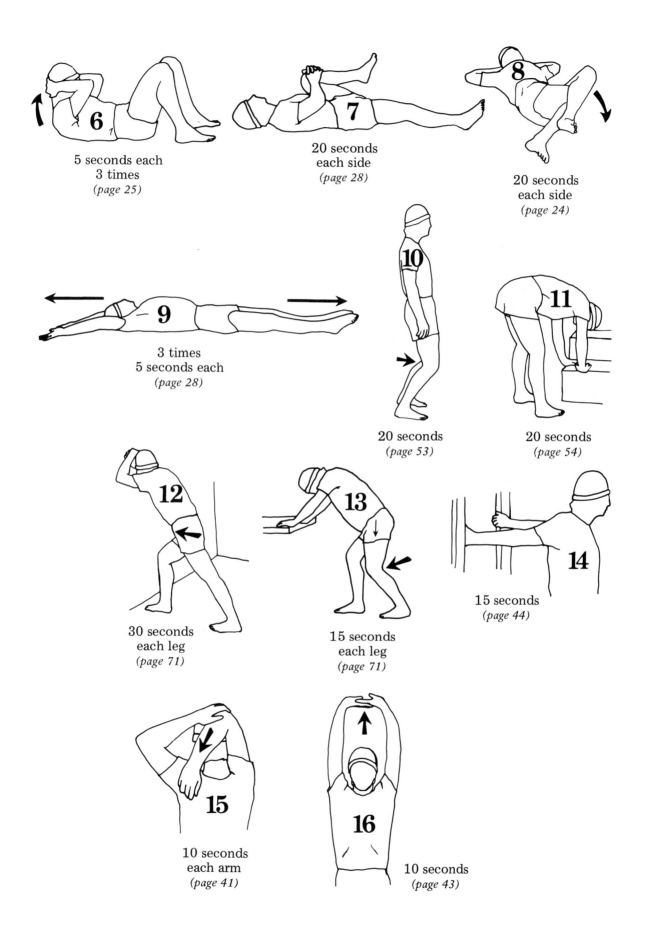

6
5 seconds each
3 times
(page 25)

7
20 seconds
each side
(page 28)

8
20 seconds
each side
(page 24)

9
3 times
5 seconds each
(page 28)

10
20 seconds
(page 53)

11
20 seconds
(page 54)

12
30 seconds
each leg
(page 71)

13
15 seconds
each leg
(page 71)

14
15 seconds
(page 44)

15
10 seconds
each arm
(page 41)

16
10 seconds
(page 43)

Before & After

Indoor and Outdoor Work

Approximately 5 Minutes

Before you do any indoor or outdoor work such as cleaning, painting, gardening, digging, building, carrying heavy loads, do a few minutes of easy stretching. This will help get your body ready to work efficiently without the usual muscle tightness and stiffness that results from this kind of work. Stretch to reduce muscle tension and make work easier.

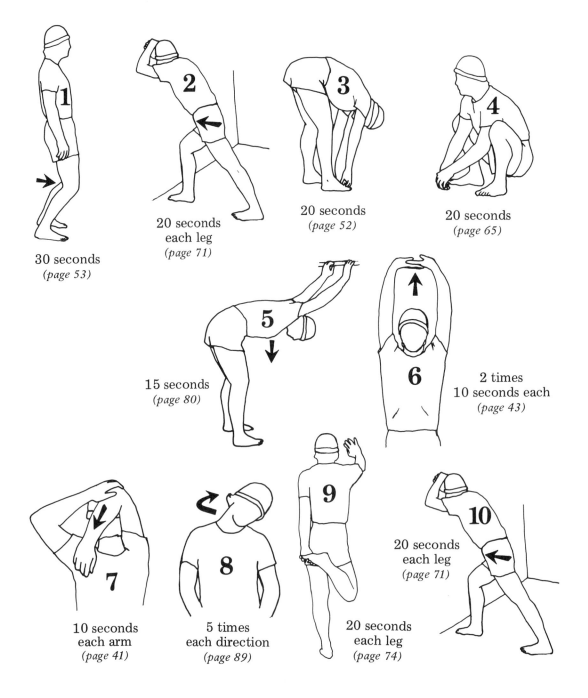

30 seconds
(page 53)

20 seconds
each leg
(page 71)

20 seconds
(page 52)

20 seconds
(page 65)

15 seconds
(page 80)

2 times
10 seconds each
(page 43)

10 seconds
each arm
(page 41)

5 times
each direction
(page 89)

20 seconds
each leg
(page 74)

20 seconds
each leg
(page 71)

For

Lower Back Tension

Approximately 4 Minutes

These stretches are designed for the relief of muscular low back pain and are also good for relieving tension in the upper back, shoulders and neck. For best results do them every night just before going to sleep. Hold only stretch tensions that feel good to you. *Do not overstretch.*

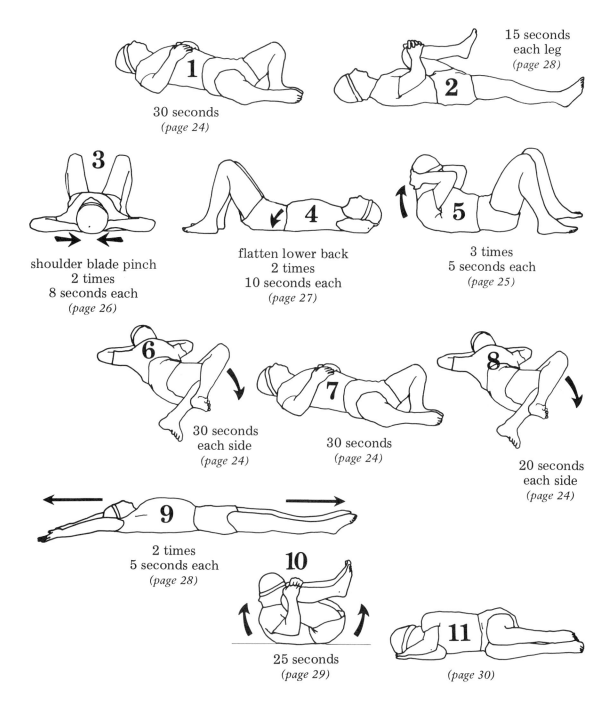

1 — 30 seconds
(page 24)

2 — 15 seconds each leg
(page 28)

3 — shoulder blade pinch
2 times
8 seconds each
(page 26)

4 — flatten lower back
2 times
10 seconds each
(page 27)

5 — 3 times
5 seconds each
(page 25)

6 — 30 seconds each side
(page 24)

7 — 30 seconds
(page 24)

8 — 20 seconds each side
(page 24)

9 — 2 times
5 seconds each
(page 28)

10 — 25 seconds
(page 29)

11 — *(page 30)*

After
Sitting
Approximately 5 Minutes

This is a series of stretches to do after sitting for a long time. The sitting position causes the blood to pool in the lower legs and feet, the hamstring muscles to tighten up, and the back and neck muscles to become stiff and tight. These stretches will improve your circulation and loosen up those areas that are tense from a prolonged period of sitting.

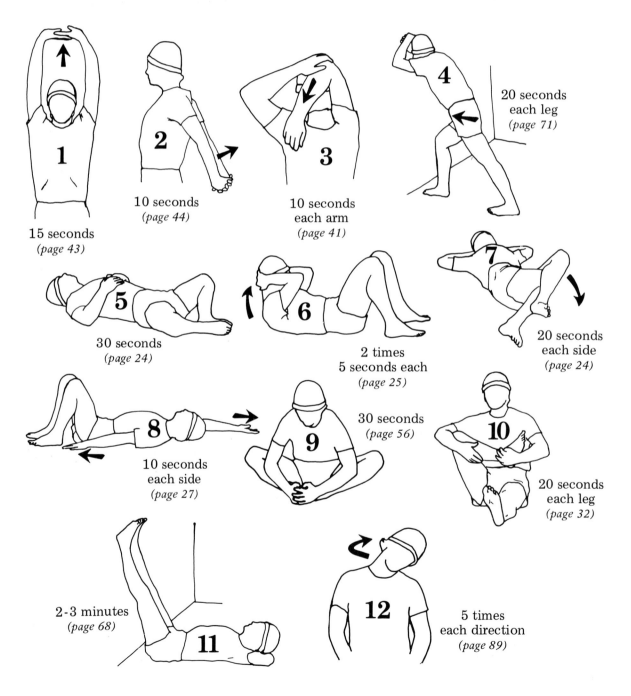

1
15 seconds
(page 43)

2
10 seconds
(page 44)

3
10 seconds
each arm
(page 41)

4
20 seconds
each leg
(page 71)

5
30 seconds
(page 24)

6
2 times
5 seconds each
(page 25)

7
20 seconds
each side
(page 24)

8
10 seconds
each side
(page 27)

9
30 seconds
(page 56)

10
20 seconds
each leg
(page 32)

11
2-3 minutes
(page 68)

12
5 times
each direction
(page 89)

While Watching

TV

Many people think they don't have enough time to stretch, yet watch several hours of television a night. If you want to help yourself, stretch as you watch TV. This will not interfere with your viewing and you will be accomplishing something during otherwise sedentary times.

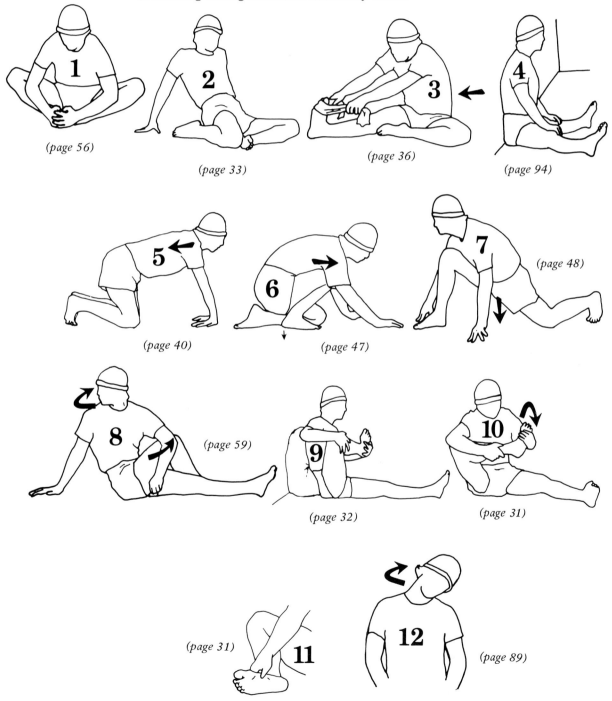

1 *(page 56)*

2 *(page 33)*

3 *(page 36)*

4 *(page 94)*

5 *(page 40)*

6 *(page 47)*

7 *(page 48)*

8 *(page 59)*

9 *(page 32)*

10 *(page 31)*

11 *(page 31)*

12 *(page 89)*

Spontaneous Stretches

You can't say you don't have time to stretch. Reading a
paper, talking on the phone, waiting for a bus . . . these are
times for easy, relaxed stretching. Be creative; think of
stretches to do during normally wasted time.

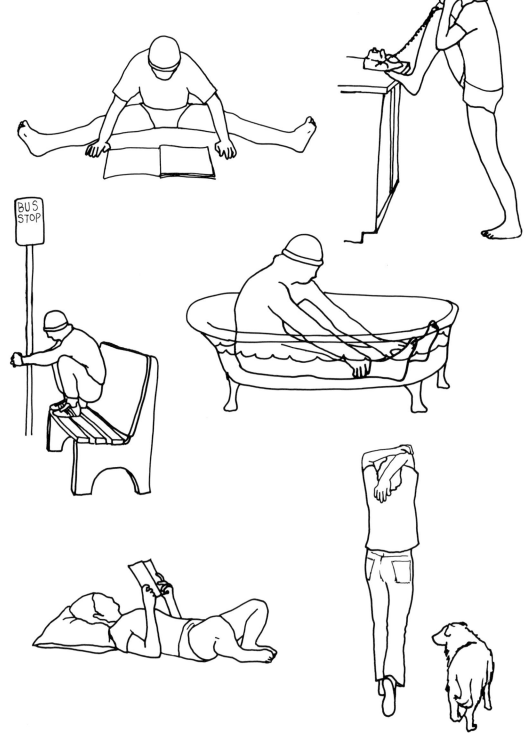

Stretching Routines: Sports and Activities

These routines will help prepare you for various sports and activities. Each routine has general stretches for the whole body, as well as specific stretches for that particular sport or activity.

To begin with, follow these routines, but after a while, you may want to develop your own routines. This is all right to do, *so long as you follow the correct method of stretching* (see pp. 12-20). Be sure you know the individual stretches before you do the routines. For instructions, refer to the page number below each drawing.

To Teachers and Coaches: These routines can serve as guidelines. You may wish to change some part of the routines to meet specific needs and time allotments.

Before and After
Baseball/Softball
Approximately 12 Minutes

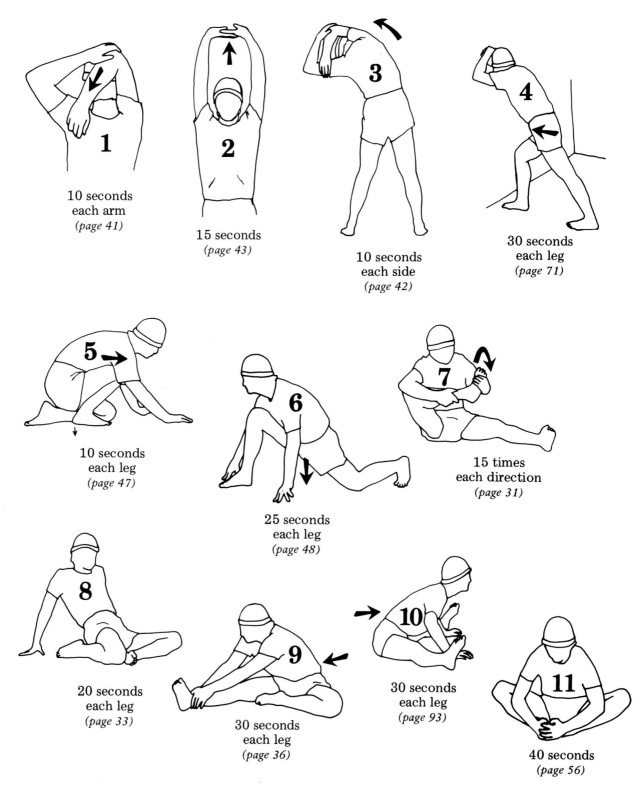

10 seconds
each arm
(page 41)

15 seconds
(page 43)

10 seconds
each side
(page 42)

30 seconds
each leg
(page 71)

10 seconds
each leg
(page 47)

25 seconds
each leg
(page 48)

15 times
each direction
(page 31)

20 seconds
each leg
(page 33)

30 seconds
each leg
(page 36)

30 seconds
each leg
(page 93)

40 seconds
(page 56)

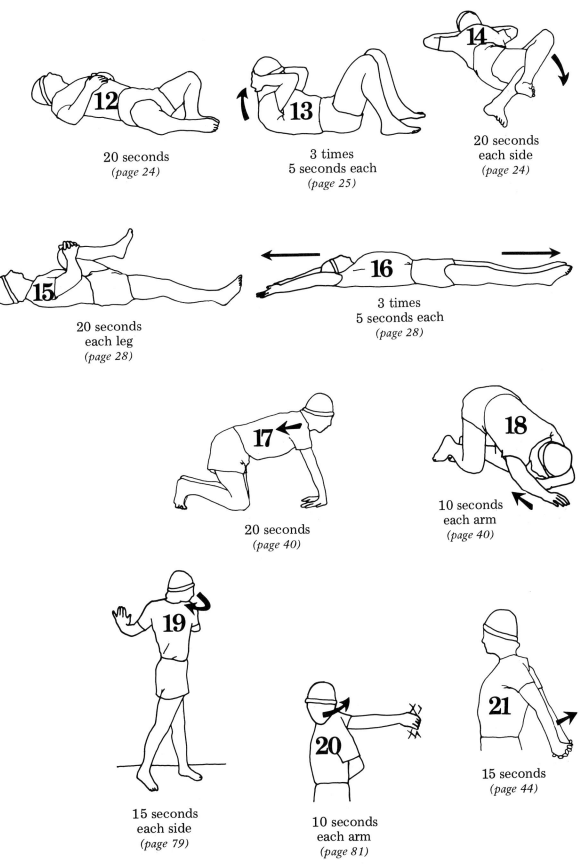

12

20 seconds
(*page 24*)

13

3 times
5 seconds each
(*page 25*)

14

20 seconds
each side
(*page 24*)

15

20 seconds
each leg
(*page 28*)

16

3 times
5 seconds each
(*page 28*)

17

20 seconds
(*page 40*)

18

10 seconds
each arm
(*page 40*)

19

15 seconds
each side
(*page 79*)

20

10 seconds
each arm
(*page 81*)

21

15 seconds
(*page 44*)

Before and After

Basketball

Approximately 12 Minutes

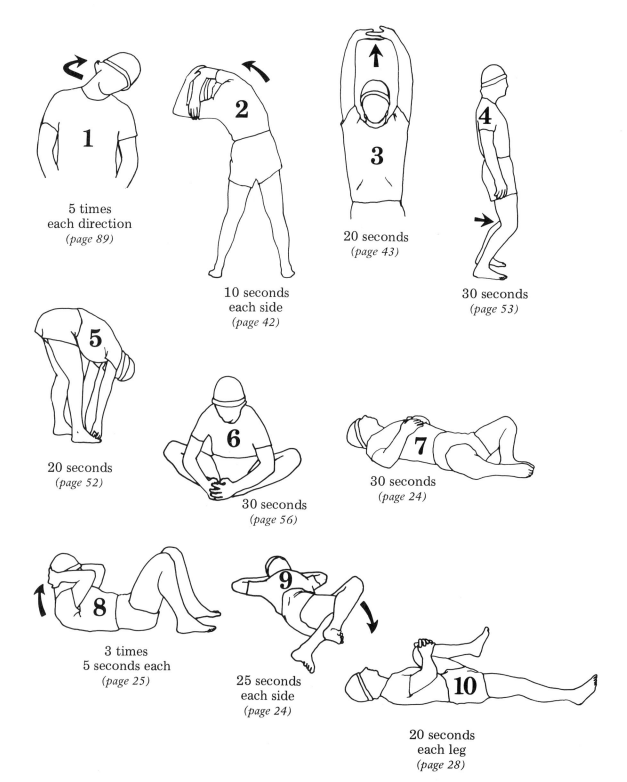

5 times
each direction
(page 89)

10 seconds
each side
(page 42)

20 seconds
(page 43)

30 seconds
(page 53)

20 seconds
(page 52)

30 seconds
(page 56)

30 seconds
(page 24)

3 times
5 seconds each
(page 25)

25 seconds
each side
(page 24)

20 seconds
each leg
(page 28)

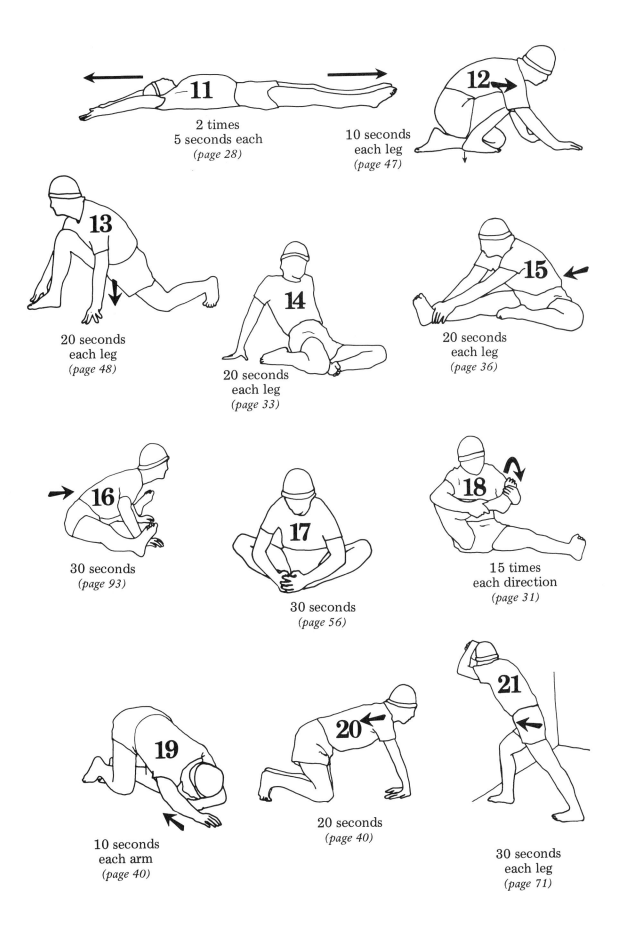

11
2 times
5 seconds each
(page 28)

12
10 seconds
each leg
(page 47)

13
20 seconds
each leg
(page 48)

14
20 seconds
each leg
(page 33)

15
20 seconds
each leg
(page 36)

16
30 seconds
(page 93)

17
30 seconds
(page 56)

18
15 times
each direction
(page 31)

19
10 seconds
each arm
(page 40)

20
20 seconds
(page 40)

21
30 seconds
each leg
(page 71)

Before and After

Cycling

Approximately 10 Minutes

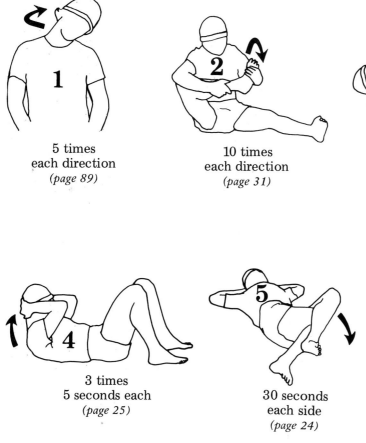

5 times
each direction
(page 89)

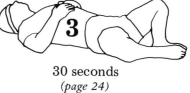

10 times
each direction
(page 31)

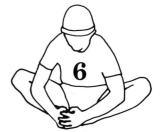

30 seconds
(page 24)

3 times
5 seconds each
(page 25)

30 seconds
each side
(page 24)

30 seconds
(page 56)

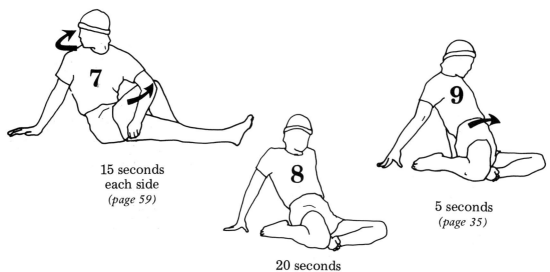

15 seconds
each side
(page 59)

20 seconds
(page 33)

5 seconds
(page 35)

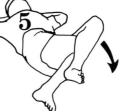

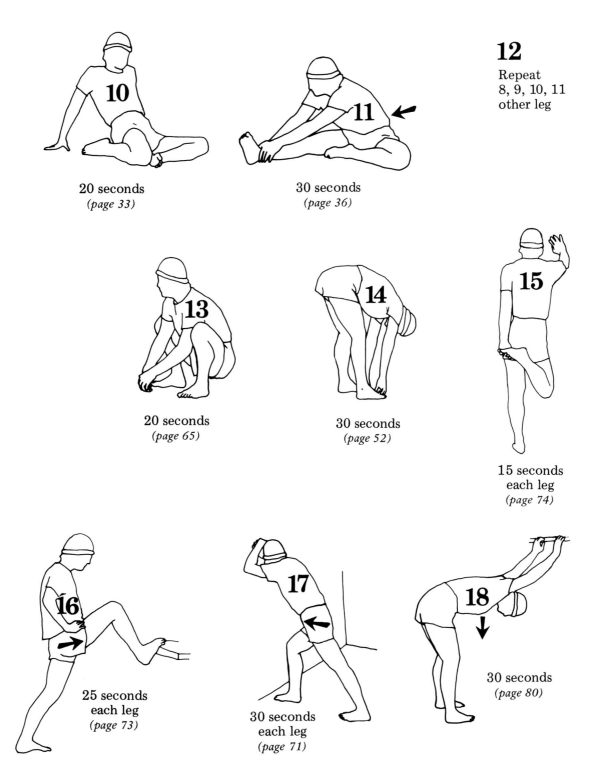

10
20 seconds
(page 33)

11
30 seconds
(page 36)

12
Repeat
8, 9, 10, 11
other leg

13
20 seconds
(page 65)

14
30 seconds
(page 52)

15
15 seconds
each leg
(page 74)

16
25 seconds
each leg
(page 73)

17
30 seconds
each leg
(page 71)

18
30 seconds
(page 80)

Before and After

Football/Rugby

Approximately 10 Minutes

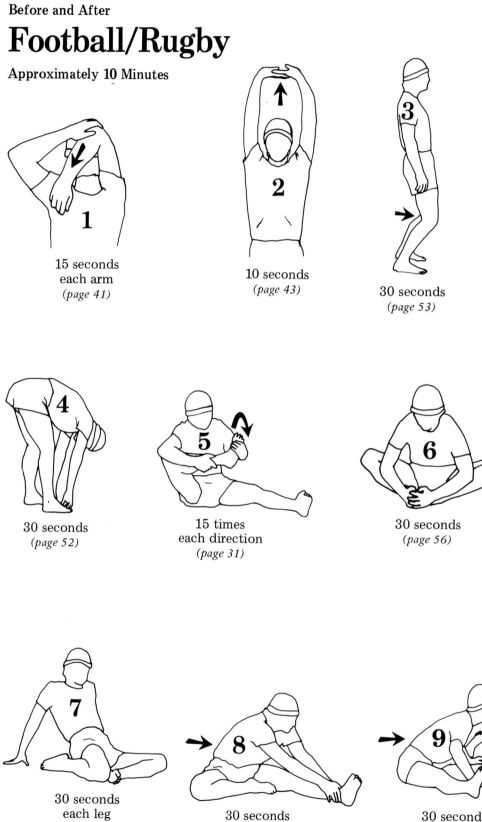

1
15 seconds
each arm
(page 41)

2
10 seconds
(page 43)

3
30 seconds
(page 53)

4
30 seconds
(page 52)

5
15 times
each direction
(page 31)

6
30 seconds
(page 56)

7
30 seconds
each leg
(page 33)

8
30 seconds
each leg
(page 36)

9
30 seconds
(page 93)

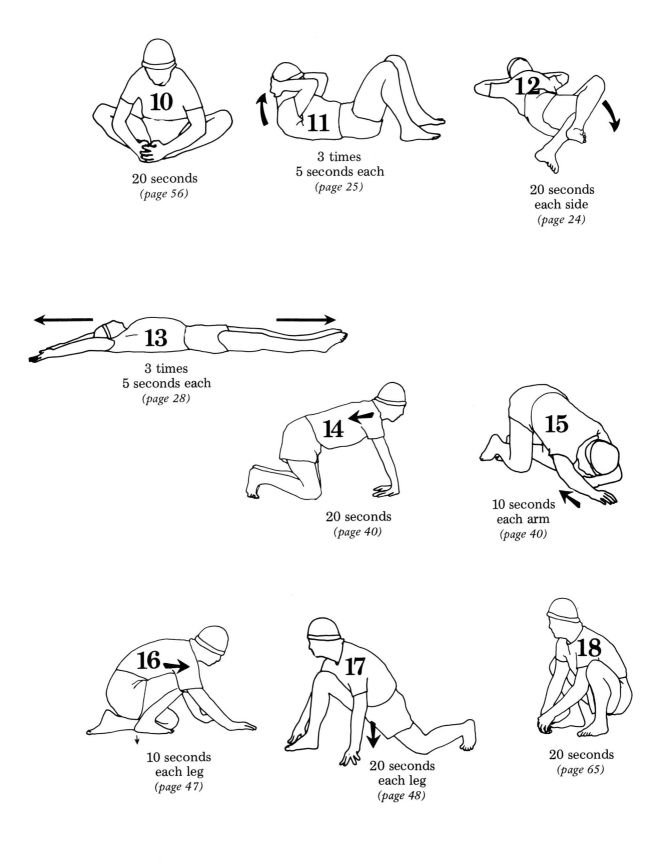

10

20 seconds
(page 56)

11

3 times
5 seconds each
(page 25)

12

20 seconds
each side
(page 24)

13

3 times
5 seconds each
(page 28)

14

20 seconds
(page 40)

15

10 seconds
each arm
(page 40)

16

10 seconds
each leg
(page 47)

17

20 seconds
each leg
(page 48)

18

20 seconds
(page 65)

Before and After

Golf

Approximately 6 Minutes

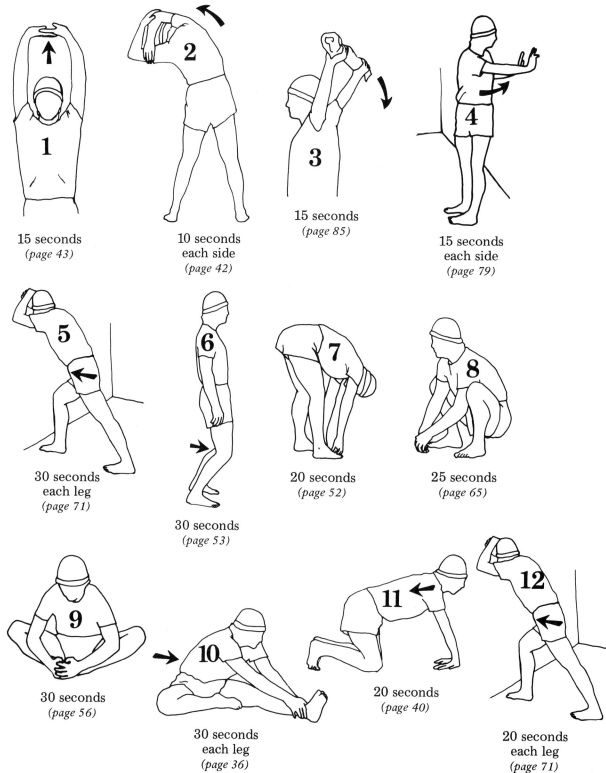

15 seconds
(*page 43*)

10 seconds
each side
(*page 42*)

15 seconds
(*page 85*)

15 seconds
each side
(*page 79*)

30 seconds
each leg
(*page 71*)

30 seconds
(*page 53*)

20 seconds
(*page 52*)

25 seconds
(*page 65*)

30 seconds
(*page 56*)

30 seconds
each leg
(*page 36*)

20 seconds
(*page 40*)

20 seconds
each leg
(*page 71*)

Before and After

Gymnastics/
Figure Skating/Dance

Approximately 15 Minutes

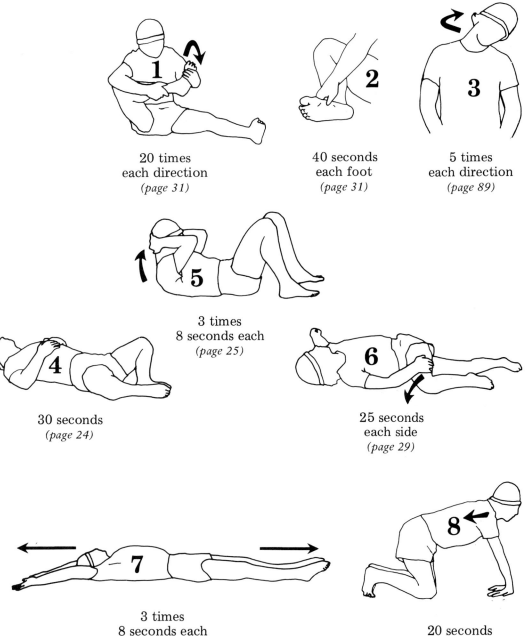

20 times
each direction
(page 31)

40 seconds
each foot
(page 31)

5 times
each direction
(page 89)

3 times
8 seconds each
(page 25)

30 seconds
(page 24)

25 seconds
each side
(page 29)

3 times
8 seconds each
(page 28)

20 seconds
(page 40)

continued . . .

. . . Gymnastics/Figure Skating/Dance

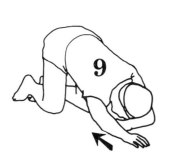

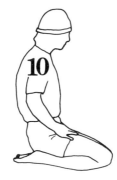

15 seconds
each arm
(page 40)

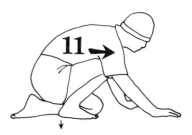

30 seconds
(page 46)

15 seconds
(page 47)

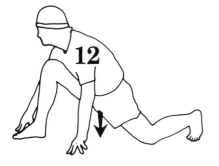

10 seconds
(page 48)

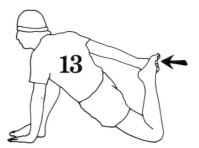

25 seconds
(page 50)

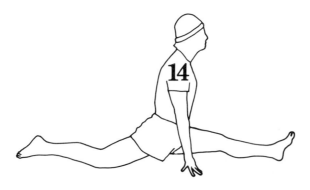

25 seconds
(page 97)

15
Repeat
11, 12, 13, 14,
other side

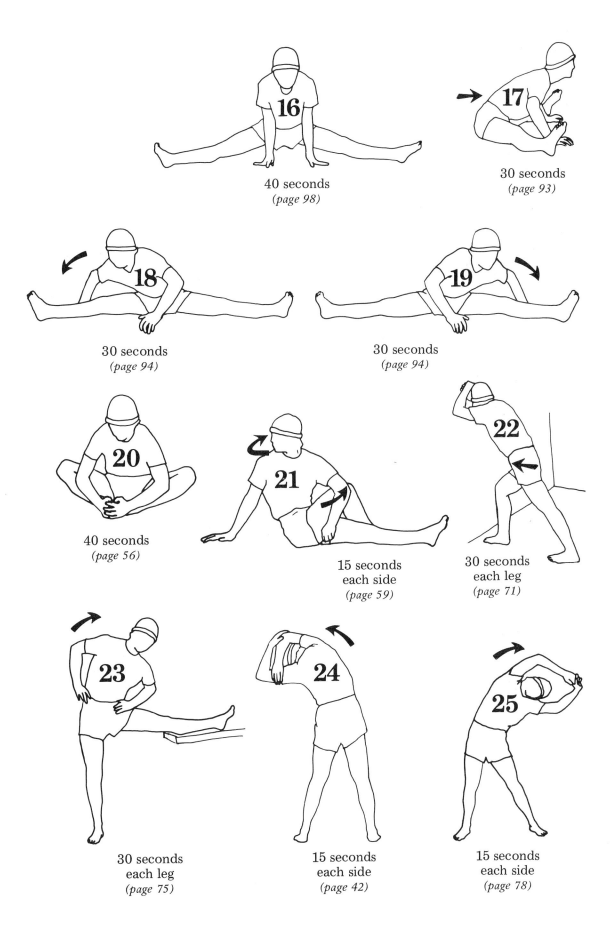

40 seconds
(page 98)

30 seconds
(page 93)

30 seconds
(page 94)

30 seconds
(page 94)

40 seconds
(page 56)

15 seconds
each side
(page 59)

30 seconds
each leg
(page 71)

30 seconds
each leg
(page 75)

15 seconds
each side
(page 42)

15 seconds
each side
(page 78)

Hiking

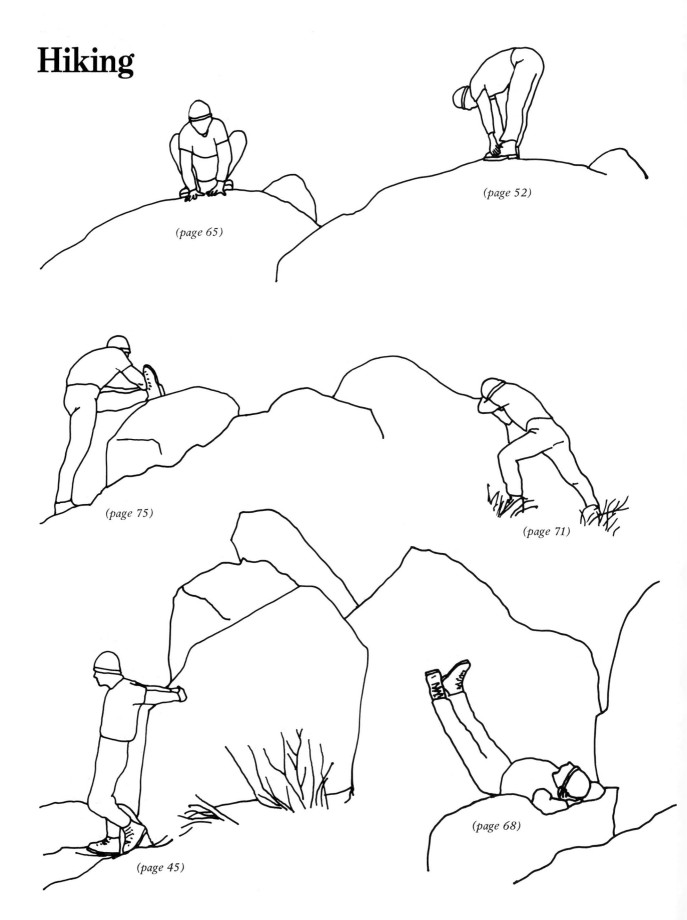

(page 52)

(page 65)

(page 75)

(page 71)

(page 68)

(page 45)

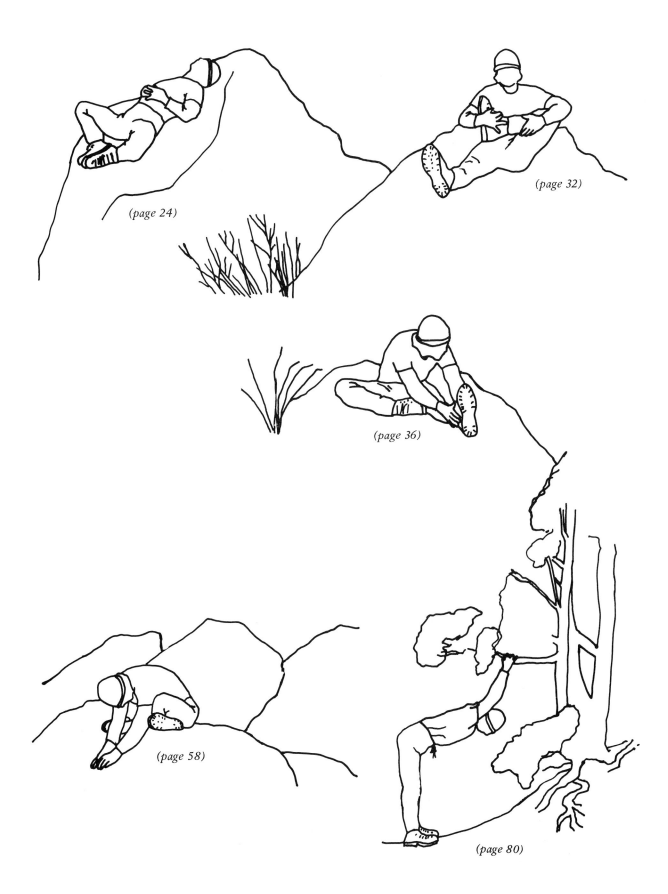

(page 24)

(page 32)

(page 36)

(page 58)

(page 80)

Before and After

Ice Hockey

Approximately 10 Minutes

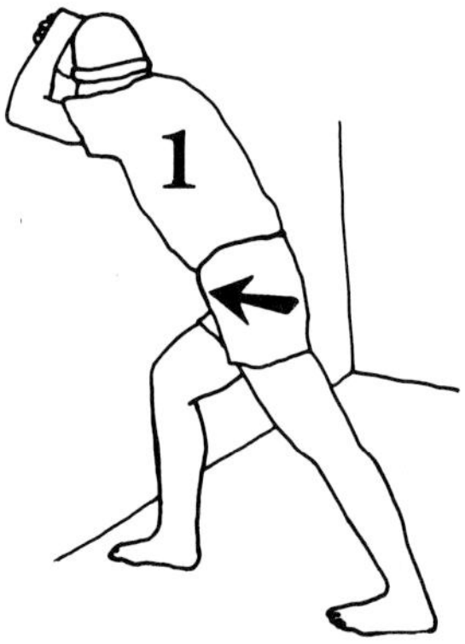

30 seconds
each leg
(page 71)

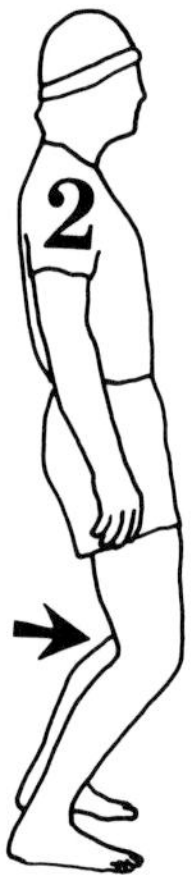

30 seconds
(page 53)

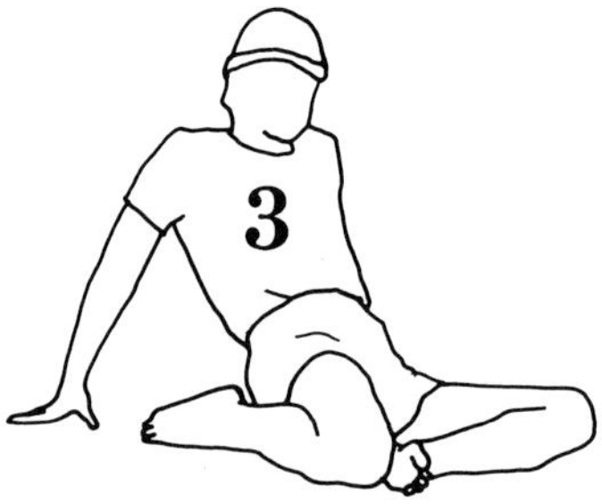

20 seconds
(page 33)

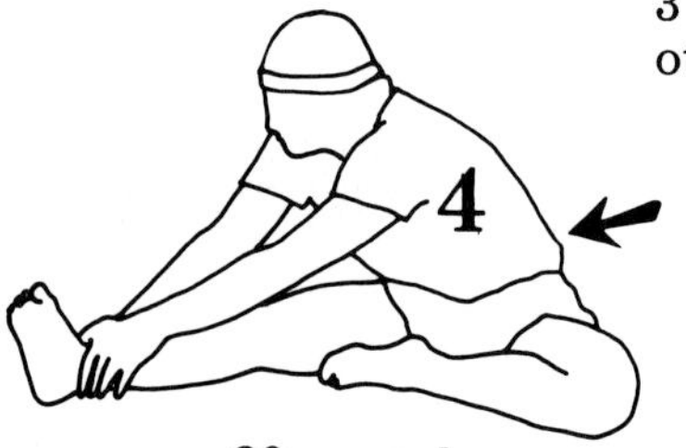

5
Repeat
3 & 4
other leg

20 seconds
(page 36)

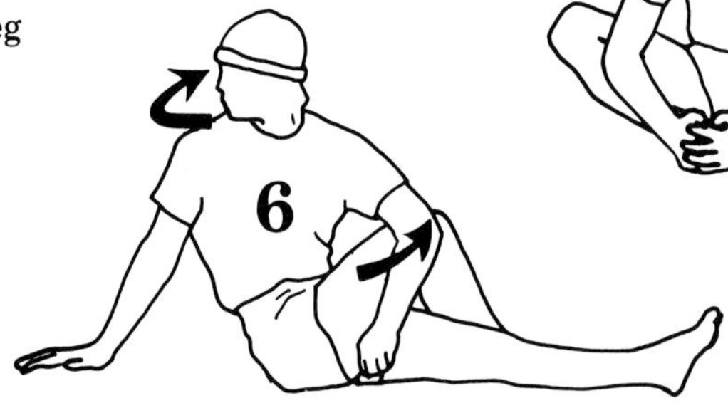

10 seconds
each side
(page 59)

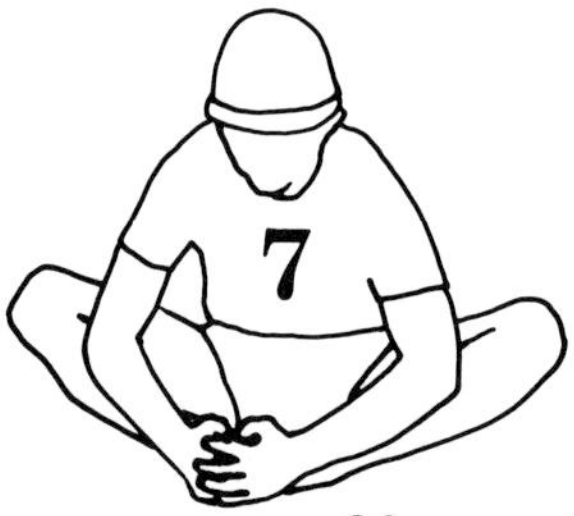

30 seconds
(page 56)

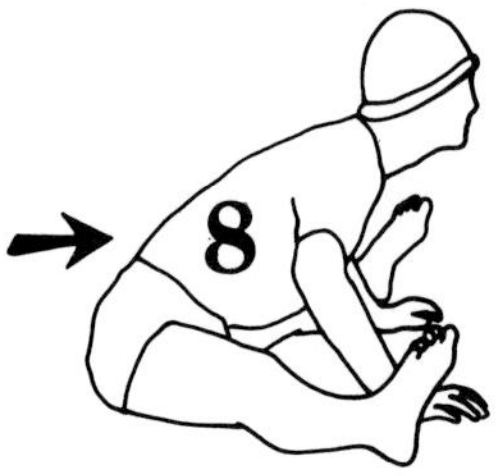

30 seconds
(page 93)

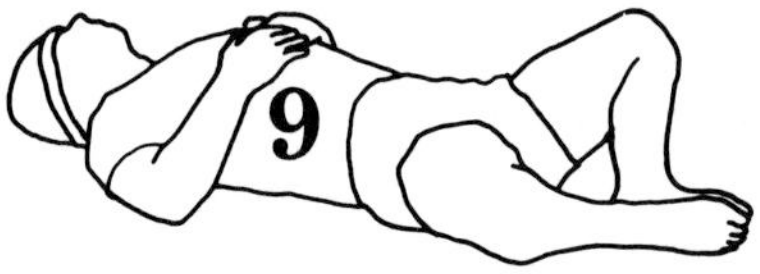

20 seconds
(page 24)

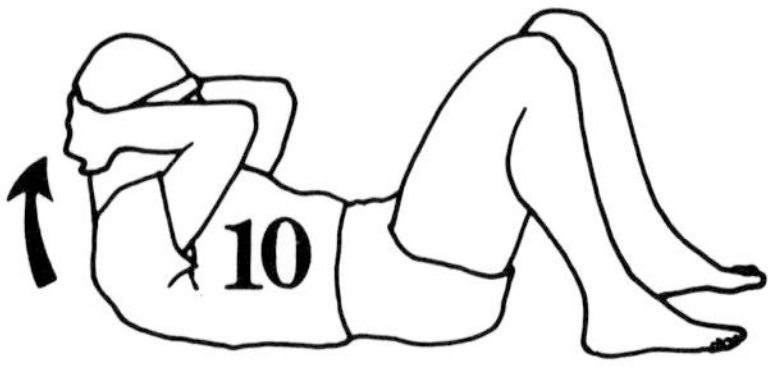

3 times
5 seconds each
(page 25)

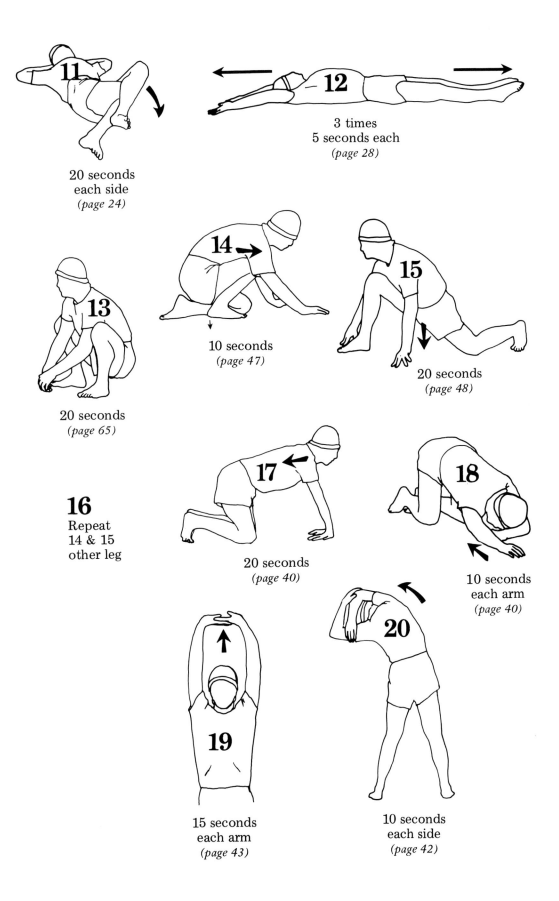

11

20 seconds
each side
(page 24)

12

3 times
5 seconds each
(page 28)

13

20 seconds
(page 65)

14

10 seconds
(page 47)

15

20 seconds
(page 48)

16
Repeat
14 & 15
other leg

17

20 seconds
(page 40)

18

10 seconds
each arm
(page 40)

19

15 seconds
each arm
(page 43)

20

10 seconds
each side
(page 42)

Before and After

Martial Arts

Approximately 17 Minutes

Note: These stretches are not intended to replace your traditional routine, but can be used for improvement of overall flexibility.

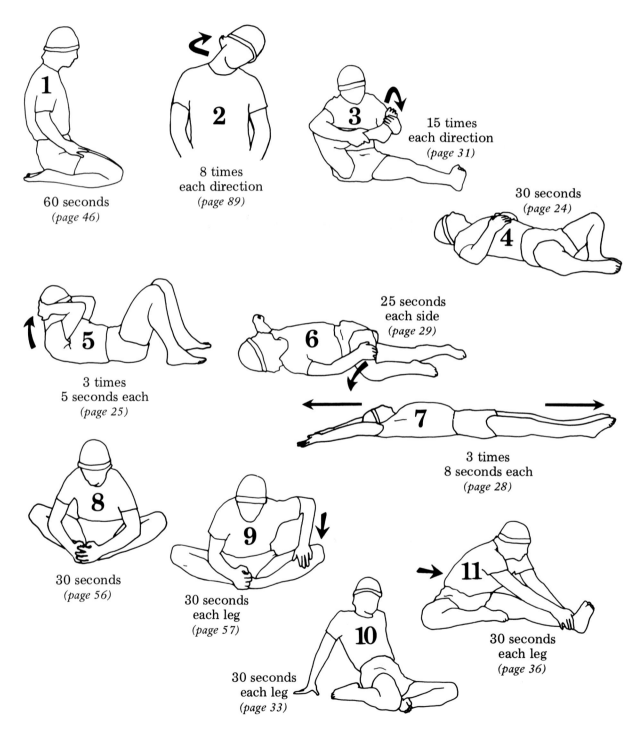

1
60 seconds
(page 46)

2
8 times
each direction
(page 89)

3
15 times
each direction
(page 31)

4
30 seconds
(page 24)

5
3 times
5 seconds each
(page 25)

6
25 seconds
each side
(page 29)

7
3 times
8 seconds each
(page 28)

8
30 seconds
(page 56)

9
30 seconds
each leg
(page 57)

10
30 seconds
each leg
(page 33)

11
30 seconds
each leg
(page 36)

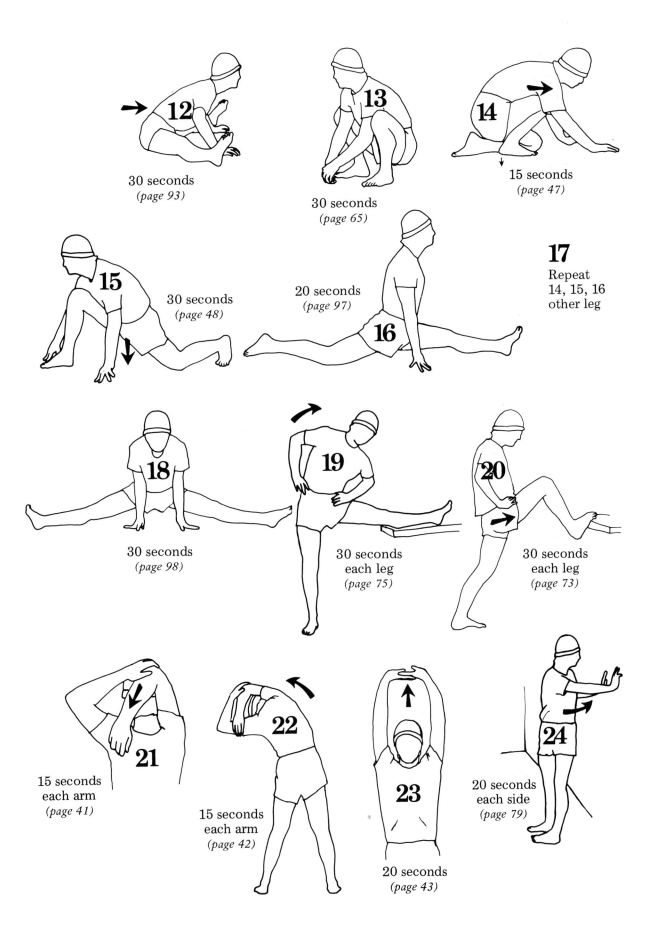

12
30 seconds
(page 93)

13
30 seconds
(page 65)

14
15 seconds
(page 47)

15
30 seconds
(page 48)

16
20 seconds
(page 97)

17
Repeat
14, 15, 16
other leg

18
30 seconds
(page 98)

19
30 seconds
each leg
(page 75)

20
30 seconds
each leg
(page 73)

21
15 seconds
each arm
(page 41)

22
15 seconds
each arm
(page 42)

23
20 seconds
(page 43)

24
20 seconds
each side
(page 79)

Before and After

Racquetball/Handball/Squash

Approximately 10 Minutes

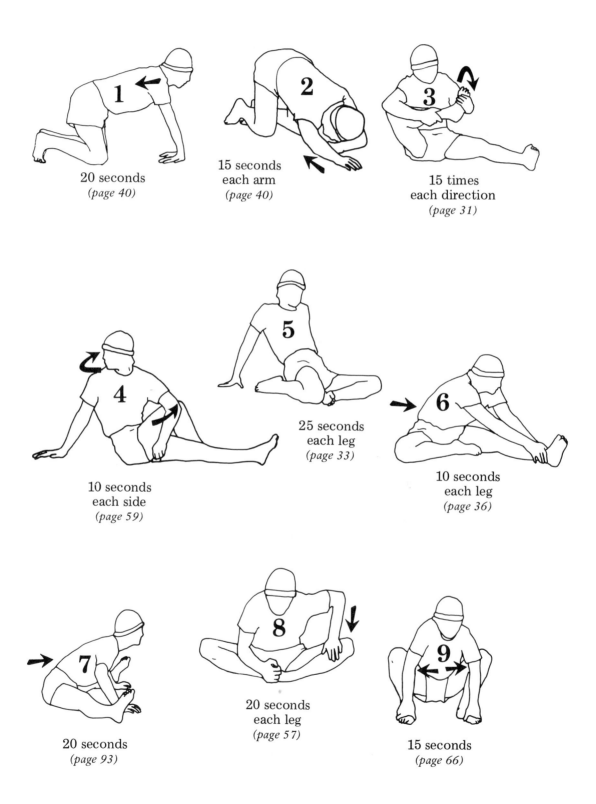

1
20 seconds
(page 40)

2
15 seconds
each arm
(page 40)

3
15 times
each direction
(page 31)

4
10 seconds
each side
(page 59)

5
25 seconds
each leg
(page 33)

6
10 seconds
each leg
(page 36)

7
20 seconds
(page 93)

8
20 seconds
each leg
(page 57)

9
15 seconds
(page 66)

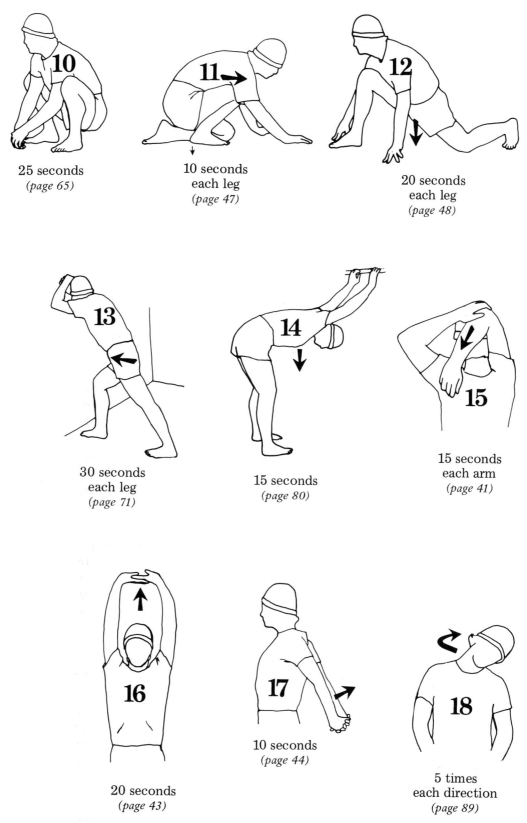

10
25 seconds
(page 65)

11
10 seconds
each leg
(page 47)

12
20 seconds
each leg
(page 48)

13
30 seconds
each leg
(page 71)

14
15 seconds
(page 80)

15
15 seconds
each arm
(page 41)

16
20 seconds
(page 43)

17
10 seconds
(page 44)

18
5 times
each direction
(page 89)

Before

Running

Approximately 9 Minutes

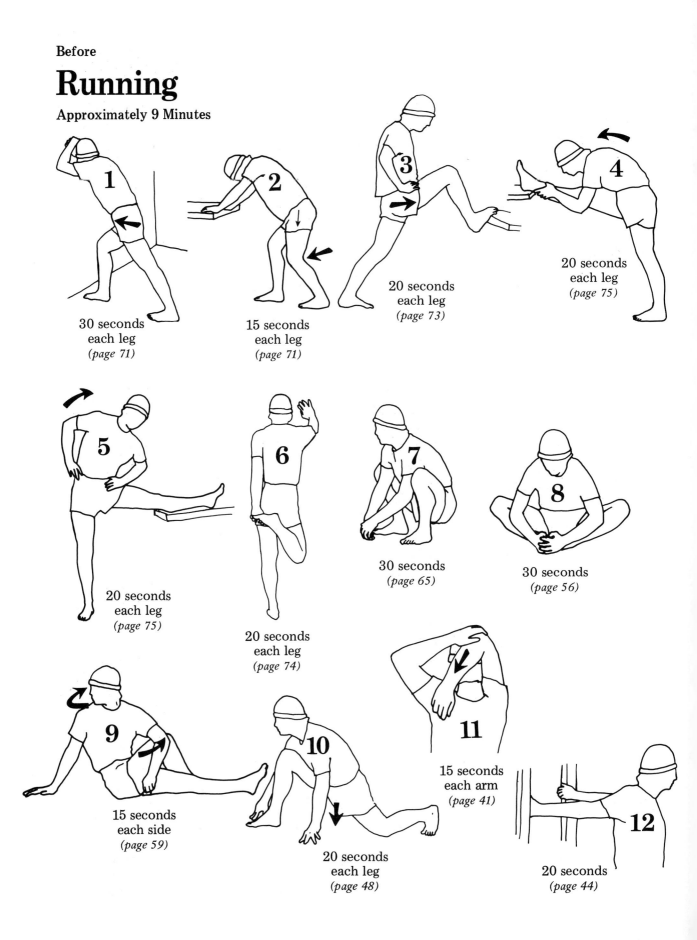

30 seconds
each leg
(page 71)

15 seconds
each leg
(page 71)

20 seconds
each leg
(page 73)

20 seconds
each leg
(page 75)

20 seconds
each leg
(page 75)

20 seconds
each leg
(page 74)

30 seconds
(page 65)

30 seconds
(page 56)

15 seconds
each side
(page 59)

20 seconds
each leg
(page 48)

15 seconds
each arm
(page 41)

20 seconds
(page 44)

After

Running

Approximately 9 Minutes

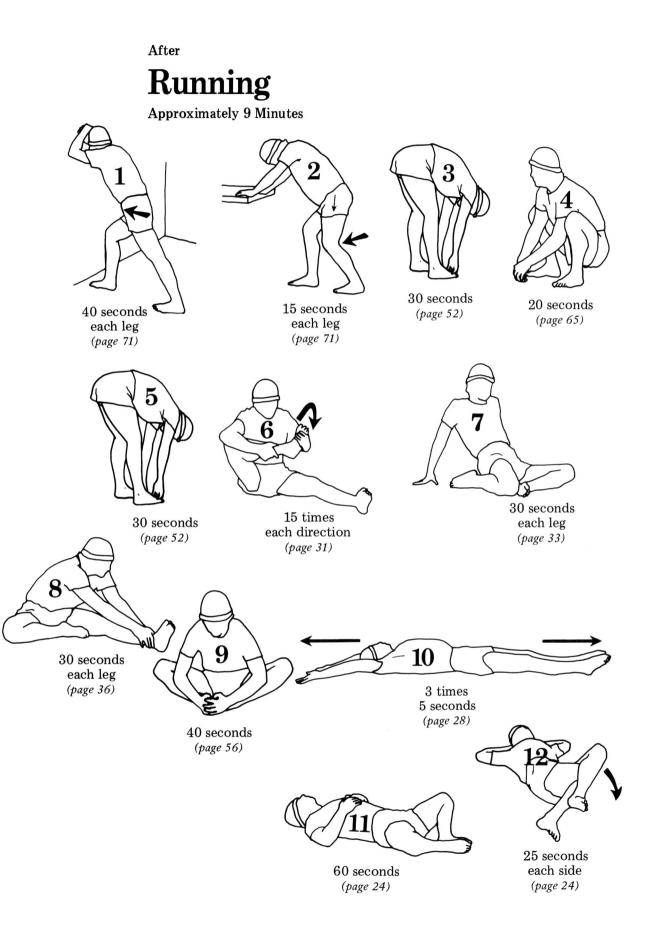

1 40 seconds each leg *(page 71)*

2 15 seconds each leg *(page 71)*

3 30 seconds *(page 52)*

4 20 seconds *(page 65)*

5 30 seconds *(page 52)*

6 15 times each direction *(page 31)*

7 30 seconds each leg *(page 33)*

8 30 seconds each leg *(page 36)*

9 40 seconds *(page 56)*

10 3 times 5 seconds *(page 28)*

11 60 seconds *(page 24)*

12 25 seconds each side *(page 24)*

Before and After
Skiing (Cross Country)
Approximately 12 Minutes

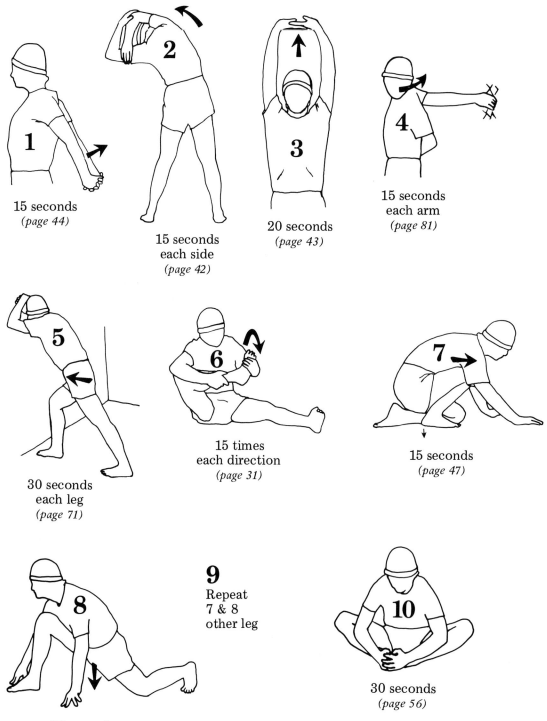

1
15 seconds
(*page 44*)

2
15 seconds
each side
(*page 42*)

3
20 seconds
(*page 43*)

4
15 seconds
each arm
(*page 81*)

5
30 seconds
each leg
(*page 71*)

6
15 times
each direction
(*page 31*)

7
15 seconds
(*page 47*)

8
30 seconds
(*page 48*)

9
Repeat
7 & 8
other leg

10
30 seconds
(*page 56*)

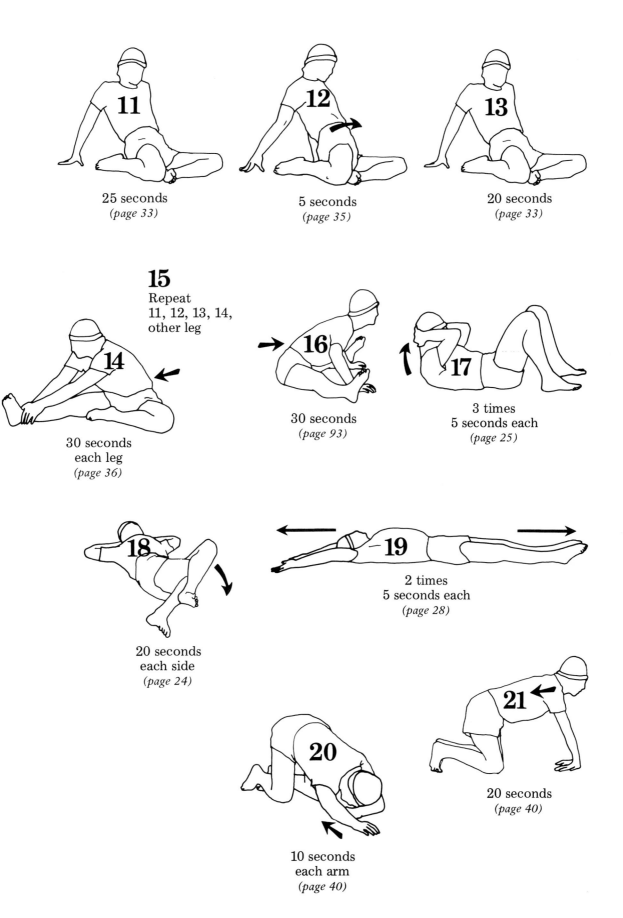

11
25 seconds
(page 33)

12
5 seconds
(page 35)

13
20 seconds
(page 33)

15
Repeat
11, 12, 13, 14,
other leg

14
30 seconds
each leg
(page 36)

16
30 seconds
(page 93)

17
3 times
5 seconds each
(page 25)

18
20 seconds
each side
(page 24)

19
2 times
5 seconds each
(page 28)

20
10 seconds
each arm
(page 40)

21
20 seconds
(page 40)

Before and After
Skiing (Downhill)
Approximately 10 Minutes

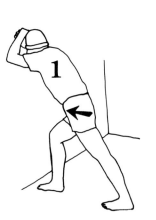
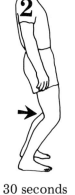
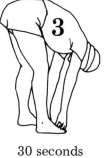
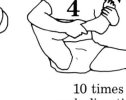
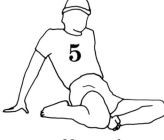
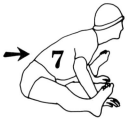

20 seconds
each leg
(page 71)

30 seconds
(page 53)

30 seconds
(page 52)

10 times
each direction
(page 31)

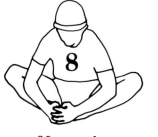
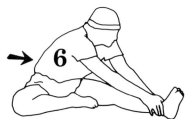
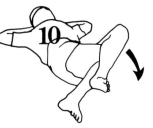

20 seconds
each leg
(page 33)

25 seconds
each leg
(page 36)

30 seconds
(page 93)

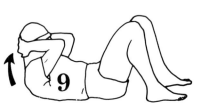

30 seconds
(page 56)

3 times
5 seconds each
(page 25)

25 seconds
each side
(page 24)

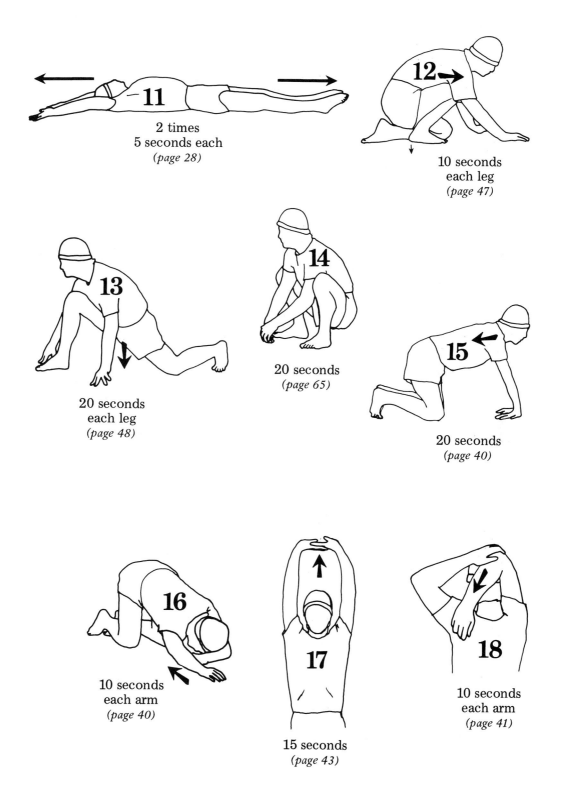

11
2 times
5 seconds each
(page 28)

12
10 seconds
each leg
(page 47)

13
20 seconds
each leg
(page 48)

14
20 seconds
(page 65)

15
20 seconds
(page 40)

16
10 seconds
each arm
(page 40)

17
15 seconds
(page 43)

18
10 seconds
each arm
(page 41)

Before and After

Soccer

Approximately 10 Minutes

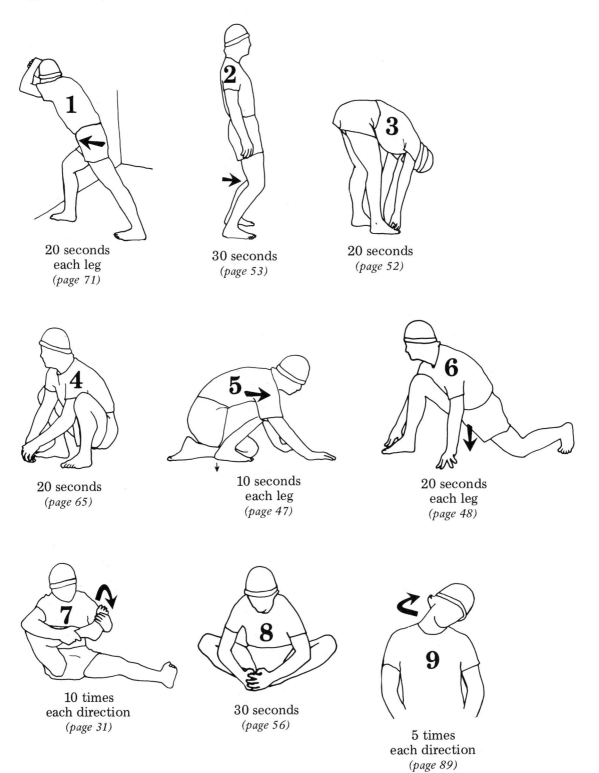

20 seconds
each leg
(page 71)

30 seconds
(page 53)

20 seconds
(page 52)

20 seconds
(page 65)

10 seconds
each leg
(page 47)

20 seconds
each leg
(page 48)

10 times
each direction
(page 31)

30 seconds
(page 56)

5 times
each direction
(page 89)

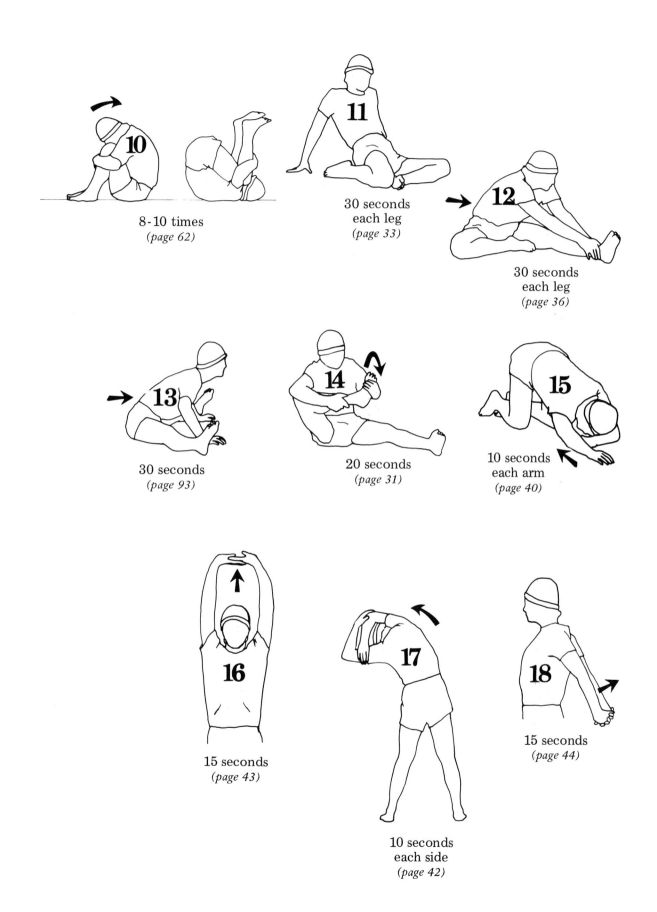

8-10 times
(page 62)

11
30 seconds
each leg
(page 33)

12
30 seconds
each leg
(page 36)

13
30 seconds
(page 93)

14
20 seconds
(page 31)

15
10 seconds
each arm
(page 40)

16
15 seconds
(page 43)

17
10 seconds
each side
(page 42)

18
15 seconds
(page 44)

Before and After

Surfing

Approximately 10 Minutes

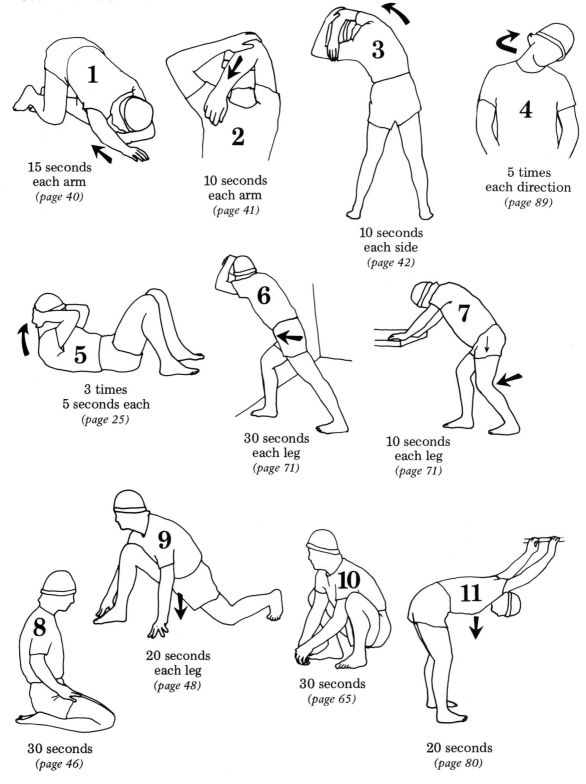

1

15 seconds
each arm
(page 40)

2

10 seconds
each arm
(page 41)

3

10 seconds
each side
(page 42)

4

5 times
each direction
(page 89)

5

3 times
5 seconds each
(page 25)

6

30 seconds
each leg
(page 71)

7

10 seconds
each leg
(page 71)

8

30 seconds
(page 46)

9

20 seconds
each leg
(page 48)

10

30 seconds
(page 65)

11

20 seconds
(page 80)

Before and After

Swimming/Water Polo

Approximately 10 Minutes

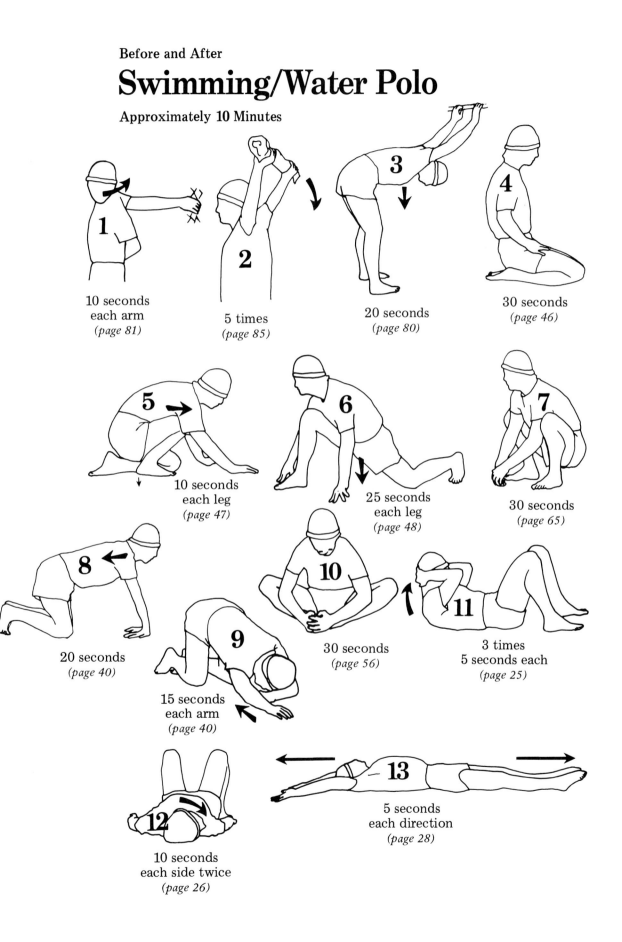

10 seconds
each arm
(page 81)

5 times
(page 85)

20 seconds
(page 80)

30 seconds
(page 46)

10 seconds
each leg
(page 47)

25 seconds
each leg
(page 48)

30 seconds
(page 65)

20 seconds
(page 40)

15 seconds
each arm
(page 40)

30 seconds
(page 56)

3 times
5 seconds each
(page 25)

10 seconds
each side twice
(page 26)

5 seconds
each direction
(page 28)

Before and After

Tennis

Approximately 12 Minutes

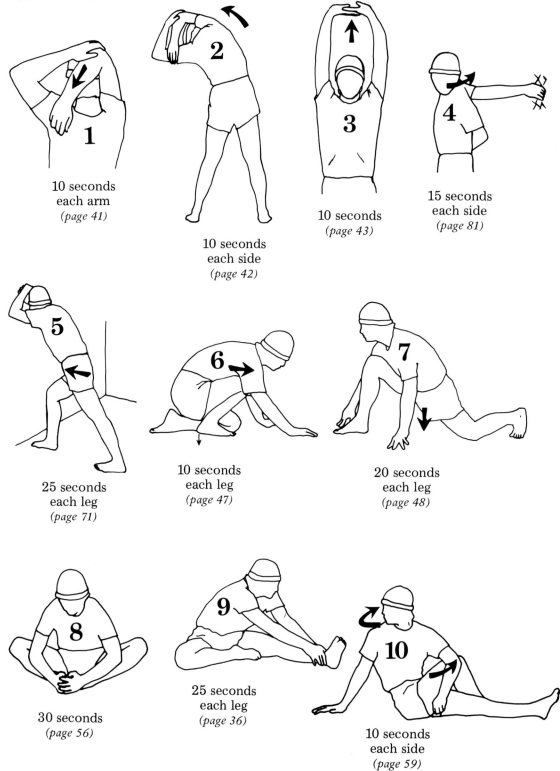

1

10 seconds
each arm
(page 41)

2

10 seconds
each side
(page 42)

3

10 seconds
(page 43)

4

15 seconds
each side
(page 81)

5

25 seconds
each leg
(page 71)

6

10 seconds
each leg
(page 47)

7

20 seconds
each leg
(page 48)

8

30 seconds
(page 56)

9

25 seconds
each leg
(page 36)

10

10 seconds
each side
(page 59)

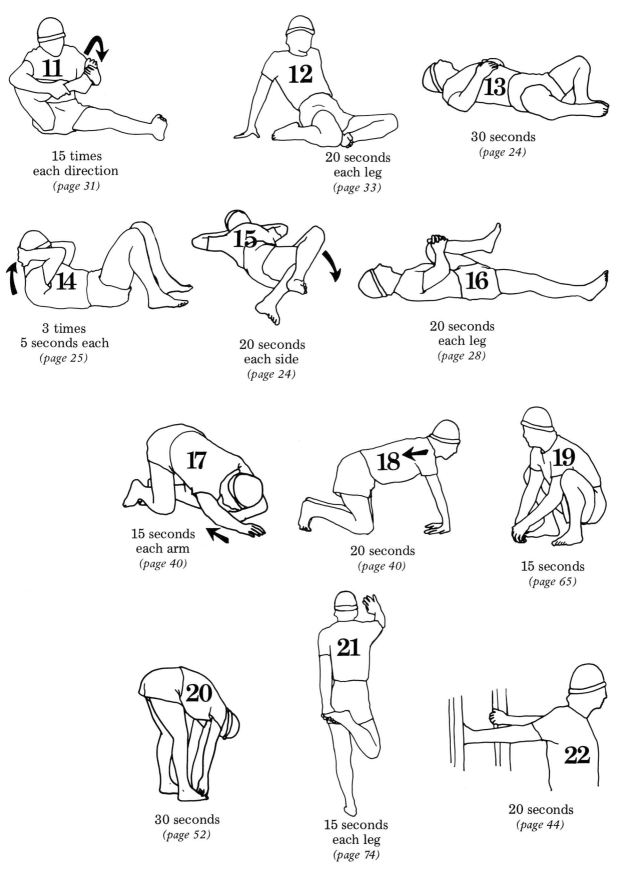

11
15 times
each direction
(page 31)

12
20 seconds
each leg
(page 33)

13
30 seconds
(page 24)

14
3 times
5 seconds each
(page 25)

15
20 seconds
each side
(page 24)

16
20 seconds
each leg
(page 28)

17
15 seconds
each arm
(page 40)

18
20 seconds
(page 40)

19
15 seconds
(page 65)

20
30 seconds
(page 52)

21
15 seconds
each leg
(page 74)

22
20 seconds
(page 44)

Before and After
Volleyball
Approximately 14 Minutes

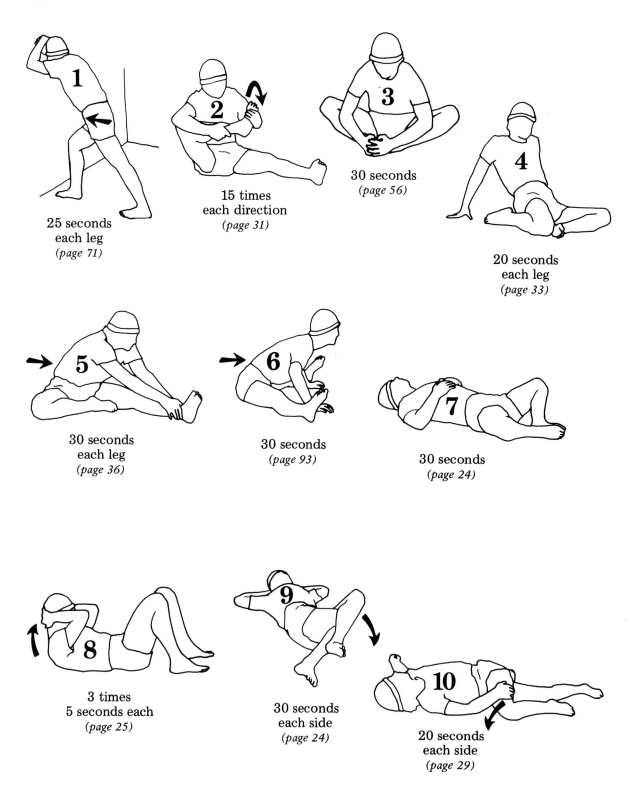

25 seconds
each leg
(page 71)

15 times
each direction
(page 31)

30 seconds
(page 56)

20 seconds
each leg
(page 33)

30 seconds
each leg
(page 36)

30 seconds
(page 93)

30 seconds
(page 24)

3 times
5 seconds each
(page 25)

30 seconds
each side
(page 24)

20 seconds
each side
(page 29)

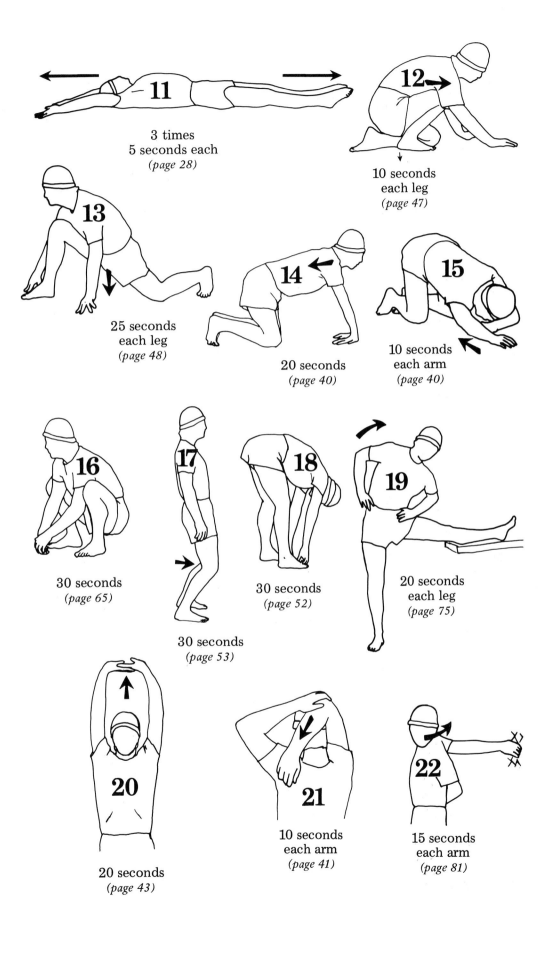

11

3 times
5 seconds each
(page 28)

12

10 seconds
each leg
(page 47)

13

25 seconds
each leg
(page 48)

14

20 seconds
(page 40)

15

10 seconds
each arm
(page 40)

16

30 seconds
(page 65)

17

30 seconds
(page 53)

18

30 seconds
(page 52)

19

20 seconds
each leg
(page 75)

20

20 seconds
(page 43)

21

10 seconds
each arm
(page 41)

22

15 seconds
each arm
(page 81)

Before and After
Weight Training
Approximately 10 Minutes

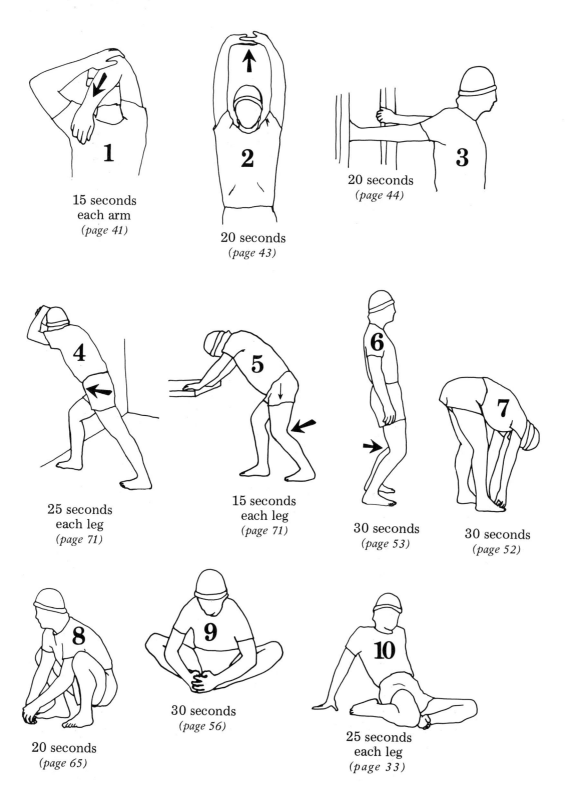

1
15 seconds
each arm
(page 41)

2
20 seconds
(page 43)

3
20 seconds
(page 44)

4
25 seconds
each leg
(page 71)

5
15 seconds
each leg
(page 71)

6
30 seconds
(page 53)

7
30 seconds
(page 52)

8
20 seconds
(page 65)

9
30 seconds
(page 56)

10
25 seconds
each leg
(page 33)

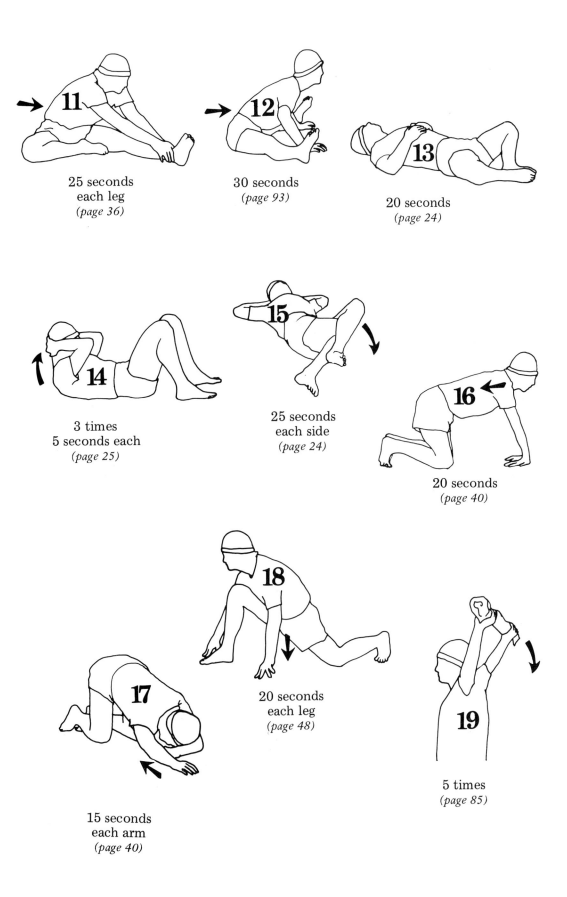

11
25 seconds
each leg
(page 36)

12
30 seconds
(page 93)

13
20 seconds
(page 24)

14
3 times
5 seconds each
(page 25)

15
25 seconds
each side
(page 24)

16
20 seconds
(page 40)

17
15 seconds
each arm
(page 40)

18
20 seconds
each leg
(page 48)

19
5 times
(page 85)

Before and After

Wrestling

Approximately 12 Minutes

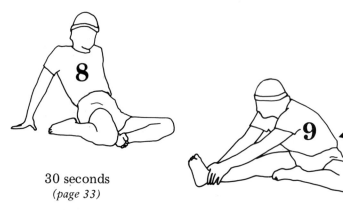

1
5 times
each direction
(page 89)

2
20 seconds
(page 43)

3
10 seconds
each side
(page 42)

4
15 seconds
(page 44)

5
10 times
each direction
(page 31)

6
25 seconds
(page 32)

7
10 seconds
(page 33)

8
30 seconds
(page 33)

9
30 seconds
(page 36)

10
Repeat
5, 6, 7, 8, 9
other leg

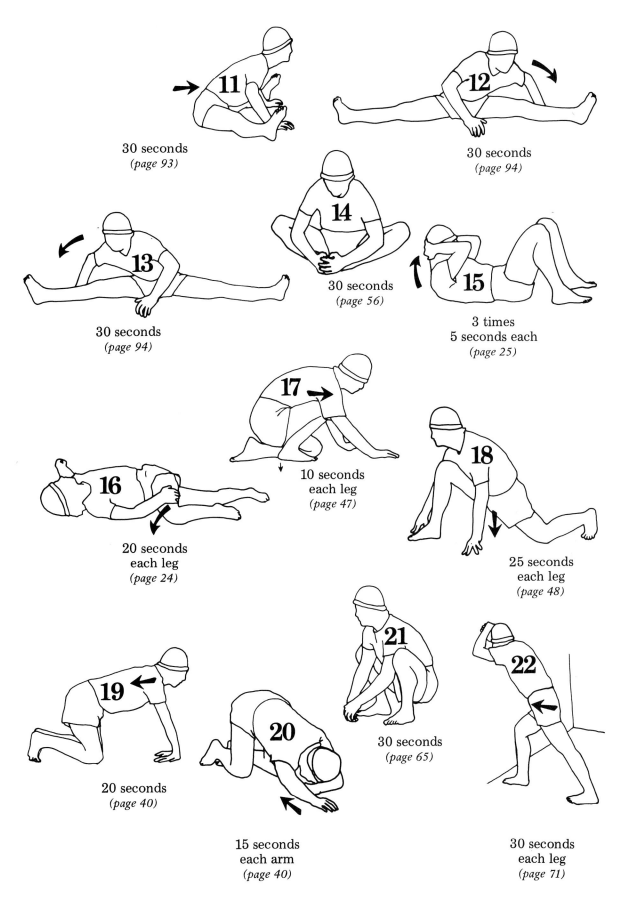

11

30 seconds
(page 93)

12

30 seconds
(page 94)

13

30 seconds
(page 94)

14

30 seconds
(page 56)

15

3 times
5 seconds each
(page 25)

16

20 seconds
each leg
(page 24)

17

10 seconds
each leg
(page 47)

18

25 seconds
each leg
(page 48)

19

20 seconds
(page 40)

20

15 seconds
each arm
(page 40)

21

30 seconds
(page 65)

22

30 seconds
each leg
(page 71)

To Teachers and Coaches

Training for student athletes has always stressed discipline, constantly pushing to new limits, and building maximum strength and power. As teacher/coaches, you are interested, of course, in team performance. But your most important goal is to educate the individuals under your supervision.

The best way to teach stretching is by your own example. When you yourself do the stretches and enjoy them, you will communicate this with your own enthusiasm. You will generate the same kind of attitude in your students.

In recent years, some attention has been given to stretching for injury prevention, but even here, there has been too much emphasis on maximum flexibility. *Stretching is entirely individual.* Let your students know that it is not a contest. There should be no comparisons made between students because each is different. The emphasis should be on the feeling of the stretch, not on how far one can go. Stressing flexibility at the beginning will only lead to overstretching, a negative attitude and possible injuries. If you notice someone who is tight or inflexible, don't single him out; emphasize the proper stretches for him alone, away from the group.

As a teacher/coach/guide, emphasize that stretching should be done with care and common sense. You do not have to set standards or push limits. Do not overwork or force your students to do too much. They will soon find what they feel good doing. They will improve naturally—and enjoy it.

It is important for people to understand that each and every one of them is an individual without comparison and with a certain potential. What it all boils down to is that all they can do is their best, nothing more.

The greatest gift you can give your students is to prepare them for the future. Teach them the value of regular exercise, of stretching daily, and of eating sensibly. Impress upon them that everyone can be fit, regardless of strength or athletic ability. Instill in your students an enthusiasm for movement and health that will last a lifetime. □

Exercises for Developing Strength

It is important for you to maintain strength throughout your life. The developmental exercises shown in the following pages will help you build and maintain strength. There are no weights involved. These exercises are based upon gaining strength and endurance through repetition and regularity.

Some of these exercises are done using total body weight. Using your own weight is not easy, so you should be patient, and gradually increase the number of sets and repetitions as you get stronger. You cannot get into shape in one day, so don't try it. Be gradual and steady, for there is no other way to improve and enjoy it. As you become regular with these exercises, you will naturally develop a good foundation of fitness.

I have included exercises for the chest and arms, for the abdominal muscles, and for the ankles and lower legs. (These ankle and lower leg exercises are good for increased running and jumping efficiency and help prevent injuries to the ankle area.) Also, I have described a stair workout that is a great supplement for total leg and knee development.

These developmental exercises are good if you are already physically active, but they are extremely important if you are just beginning to exercise, or if you have taken a long lay-off from physical activity. If you have not been physically active lately, your muscles may have become small and weak (atrophied). These exercises, coupled with regular stretching, will help greatly in restoring full use and strength to weakened muscles.

If you are a beginner, I suggest you start with strengthening the lower legs and ankles as a basic foundation of support for the entire body. The chest and arms should be gradually strengthened by doing knee push-ups. Your abdominal muscles are probably the most important muscles of your body, but often are the least developed. Learn how to strengthen your abdominals by doing these exercises on a daily basis. Your fingers, hands, wrists, and forearms can easily be strengthened by squeezing a ball.

All these exercises help strengthen the joints needed for free and easy movement. Supplement your physical activity, whether it be running, cycling, walking, swimming, tennis, racquetball, basketball, or whatever, with these developmental exercises.

EXERCISES FOR THE ABDOMINAL MUSCLES:

The abdominal muscles are the strength center of the body. They are essential for endurance. They help keep your back free from pain, assist in proper movement, easy elimination of waste, in rhythmical breathing, and in standing erect. But few of us have ever felt the energy that goes with strong abdominals.

"Sit-ups" are generally considered the best exercise for strengthening abdominal muscles. Yet sit-ups offer little in the way of rhythm and can cause severe strain. Because of this, many people understandably detest sit-ups.

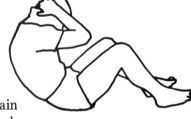

The straight legged sit-up is potentially dangerous for the lower back for this reason: your abdominal muscles can raise your body off the floor to about a 30° angle. To raise any further activates the primary hip flexor muscles, which are attached to the lower back. This puts severe stress on the lower back.

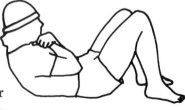

Bending your knees will relieve much of the strain in your lower back. The bent knee sit-up is good, as long as you do each sit-up fluidly and mentally concentrate on the abdominal muscles. Be careful of this exercise because people generally do too many repetitions, and when tired, jerk up quickly, which stresses the lower back.

The developmental exercise I do recommend for strengthening abdominals without straining the lower back is the *ab curl*. Here the upper body is curled forward no more than 30° and the lower back remains flat.

Here are three exercises and one variation that will work the upper, lower and sides of your abdominals. If your abdominals get tight doing these, just relax and straighten out your legs, put your hands over your head and reach in the opposite direction with a controlled stretch. Hold for 5-8 seconds. This should stretch the abdominals and relieve any tightness that might occur.

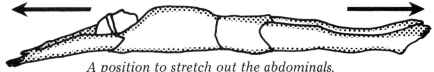

A position to stretch out the abdominals.

The Abdominal Curl (Ab Curl)

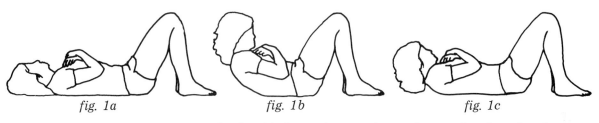

| *fig. 1a* | *fig. 1b* | *fig. 1c* |

Start on your back with knees bent and feet flat on the floor, hands across your chest (fig. 1a). Curl up, bringing your shoulder blades off the floor about 30° (fig. 1b), then lower back down to the floor (fig. 1c). Do not bob your head up and down, as this may strain your neck. Keep your head in a fixed position. Concentrate on the *upper abdominals* (solar plexis area), curling your upper body forward with your chin close to your chest (fig 1b). When you lower, or uncurl your upper body, the back of your head should not touch the floor because you are holding your chin near your chest (fig. 1c).

Do the ab curl at medium speed. Try 5 to 10. Concentrate on the muscles being used and on developing body rhythm.

The Elbow-Knee Ab Curl

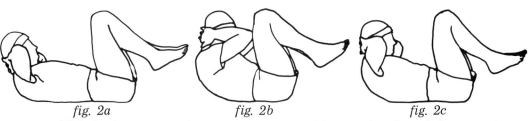

| *fig. 2a* | *fig. 2b* | *fig. 2c* |

This is done from the same starting position as the ab curl, but you interlace your fingers behind your head about ear level and raise your feet off the floor. Using your abdominal muscles, hold your upper body at about a 30° angle off the floor (fig. 2a). Now, bring your elbows forward, touching about 1-2 inches above the knees (fig. 2b). Uncurl as in fig. 2c, then raise your elbows and knees again as in fig. 2b. Your lower back should be flat at all times during these abdominal exercises.

Do this at medium speed to develop rhythm and strength. Do about 10. This works your lower and upper abdominals simultaneously.

The Alternating Elbow-Knee Ab Curl

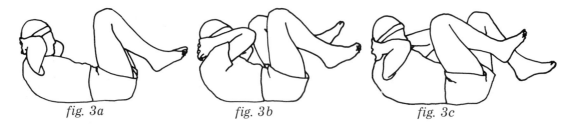

<table>
<tr><td>fig. 3a</td><td>fig. 3b</td><td>fig. 3c</td></tr>
</table>

fig. 3a   *fig. 3b*   *fig. 3c*

The starting position is the same as for the elbow-knee ab curl. Raise your shoulder blades off the mat (fig. 3a) and alternate touching your right elbow to your left knee (fig. 3b) and then left elbow to right knee (fig. 3c). This would be one count. Keep your upper body in a flexed position during this exercise. The direction of knee movement should be forward and back, like riding a bicycle (only with less range of motion). To be able to touch knee to opposite elbow, your upper body will be turning slightly from side to side, but don't let your knees cross the mid-line of your body. Relax your ankles while doing these last two types of ab curls. Develop rhythm as you exercise. See what 10 repetitions feel like.

I suggest you develop your upper abdominals by initially concentrating on the first ab curl described, and then slowly work on the other two types and the variation shown below. Develop rhythm, strength and coordination. The last two exercises take more strength and coordination than the first. Start doing these for 3-5 minutes at a time, going from one exercise to another. Strong abdominals are extremely important for your health.

Variation of the Ab Curl

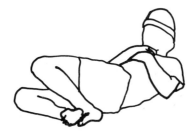

Lean your knees off to the right side. Pull your upper body forward, thinking of your chin going directly toward the top of your left hip. Concentrate on curling up, using your left side abdominal muscles. Be sure to keep chin close to chest; do not move your head up and down during the exercise. This exercise is tougher than it might look. Try 5 to 10, each side. □

EXERCISES FOR ARMS AND CHEST

Knee push-ups are very good for upper body development and maintaining muscle tone. They can be done in different ways to work different parts of the arms and upper body, without putting a strain on the lower back.

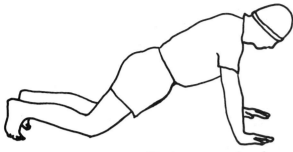

Start on your hands and knees, with hands parallel to each other and a little more than shoulder-width apart. The wider apart your hands are, the more you work your chest (pectoral muscles).

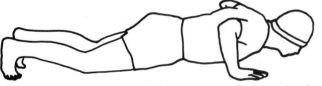

Lower your body straight down until you barely touch your chest to the floor, then push yourself straight up to the starting position (first drawing above).

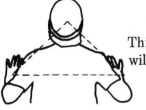

Think of a triangle, with a line drawn between your chin and two hands. This will keep your back straight and your butt from sticking up in the air.

To develop the back of your upper arms (triceps), place your hands about shoulder-width apart and keep your elbows close to your body. Don't let your elbows bow out, but keep them directly over your hands and next to the sides of your upper body. This is an isolation exercise for the triceps.

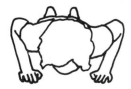

To develop triceps

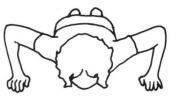

To develop pectorals

Variation: Do push-ups on finger tips.

After doing push-ups, stretching in any of these positions below feels good:

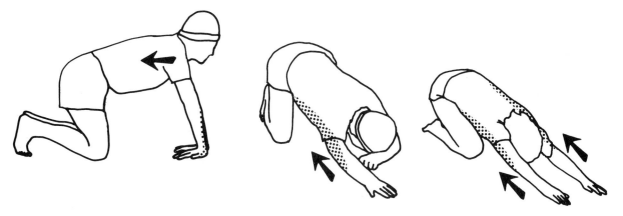

Knee push-ups are great for both men and women. When done properly and in sufficient numbers they are extremely good for developing the chest and arms. For women they help to maintain the bustline, prevent sagging muscles, and improve muscle tone.

A Suggested Knee Push-Up Workout for a Beginner: 15 push-ups and then 15 seconds of stretching; 10 push-ups and another 15 seconds to stretch; and finally five push-ups and end the workout with a stretch for your shoulders, arms and chest. Use the previous two stretches in between the sets.

For a more advanced workout, start with 35 push-ups and work your way down, five at a time. □

EXERCISES FOR ANKLES, TOES, AND LOWER LEGS

Most exercises for strength development are for body areas above the knees. Few people concentrate on developing their toes, ankles, and lower legs.

Through necessity, I devised a series of ankle exercises to help in the rehabilitation of injured athletes. As I experimented with these exercises, I found they not only helped in recovery from ankle injuries, but could be done regularly to prevent injuries and maintain strength and coordination in the lower legs and ankles.

The following exercises help develop strength in the tendons and muscles, and aid in the development of power in the toes, ankles, and lower legs. They can be done anywhere; all you need is someone to help you.

They could help a great many older people, who need to have this part of their bodies strong for everyday use. They are excellent for people who have weak ankles, or those who want to develop stronger lower legs for specific skills. And they should also be used to help prevent or lessen the chance of shin splints. Try these exercises for a few weeks to see if they make any difference in the way your legs feel.

Phase 1: Extension of the Ankle & Dorsi-Flexion of the Foot

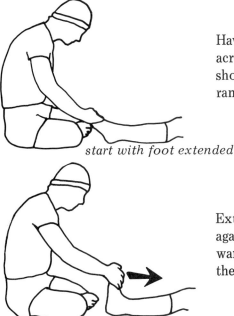

Have your partner set the palm of his right hand across your toes and on top of your left foot. He should provide *medium resistance*, so it allows full range of motion for your ankle.

start with foot extended

Extend your ankle at a medium, rhythmical pace against the resistance. By bringing your toes toward your shin (dorsi-flexing), you will be working the front of your lower leg (*anterior tibialis*).

At first do 20-25 repetitions per set. Your partner should help you by counting silently, while you concentrate on extending your ankle and dorsi-flexing your foot.

Phase 2: Flexing the Ankle and Extending the Foot

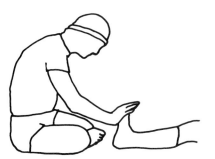

Next, have your partner place the palm of his right hand on the ball and toes of your left foot, with his thumb and index finger next to your big toe. Again, your partner should allow your ankle full range of motion, but provide enough resistance to make you concentrate. He should encourage you to use your toes as you push your foot into his hand.

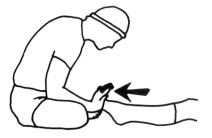

Work on flexing your toes at the end of each repetition for strength and power. Do 20-25 reps. After each movement forward, relax your ankle and foot while your partner pushes your foot quickly and gently back into the starting position.

Phase 3: Inward Movement of the Foot at Ankle Joint

Have your partner place the thumb and index finger of his right hand around the heel of your left foot. He shouldn't hold your heel, but provide a support to keep your leg and ankle fairly stable during the next two phases. The palm of his left hand should be placed on the inside of your left foot.

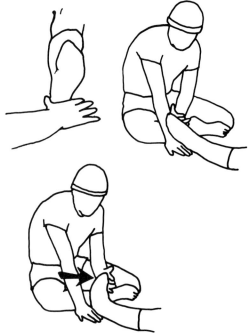

Move your foot in an inward direction, against the mild but constant pressure of his hand. Concentrate on moving at the ankle joint only. Work on a full range of motion. Develop strength. Do 20-25 reps.

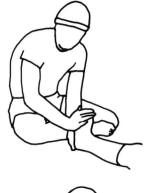

Phase 4: Outward Movement of the Foot at the Ankle Joint

Have your partner switch hands and hold the heel of your left foot with his left hand and place his right hand on the outside of your foot, with his palm just below your little toe.

Now rhythmically move your foot in an outward direction. Concentrate on moving your foot at the ankle joint. Develop rhythm, concentrating on the range of motion. Do 20-25 reps.

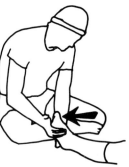

Working the ankle in all four directions is one set. Do these exercises continuously, 3-4 sets each ankle. As you become stronger, gradually increase the number of repetitions.

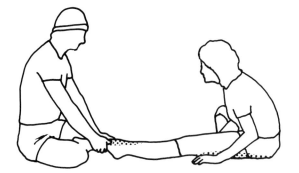

After you complete 3-4 sets of 20-25 reps each, your partner should gently extend your foot as shown below. Slowly lean forward to stretch the top of your foot. Hold a comfortable stretch for 10-20 seconds.

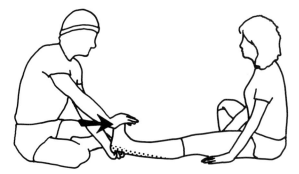

To stretch the back of the lower leg, rest your heel on the palm of your partner's hand. He should dorsiflex your foot and extend your ankle by pushing the ball of your foot toward the front of your lower leg. He will hold your foot in this position, giving a slight stretch to the calf. Hold for 15 seconds.

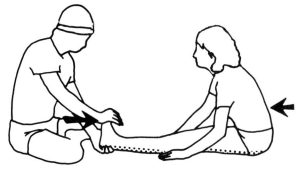

To increase the stretch, slowly bend from the hips, as your partner holds the stretch position. This should help stretch the entire leg even though you may only feel it in your calf. Get a good stretch. Do not strain. Hold 30-40 seconds. If you have sciatic nerve pain in the back of the upper thigh (hamstrings) this will help you to stretch the back of your leg without pain. Stretch only with a comfortable, controlled feeling.

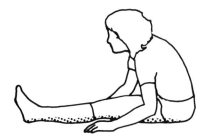

After your partner has released his hands from your foot, stretch your leg by bending forward from the hips. Now your leg should feel more flexible. Come out of each stretch position slowly. □

EXERCISES FOR FINGERS, HANDS, WRISTS, AND FOREARMS

Another developmental exercise which can be done anywhere is squeezing a ball. This strengthens fingers, hands, wrists and forearms. You need strength in these areas for many athletic activities as well as for performing everyday tasks. You can carry a rubber ball (about 2½ inches in diameter) in your pocket or in your car. Then, at normally wasted times, you can use it to develop these muscles that most of us take for granted.

There are several ways to squeeze a ball. First, squeeze it in one hand with all your fingers and thumb. Squeeze until you feel your hand tire, then squeeze a few more times.

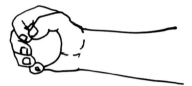

Another way is to use one finger and thumb. Start squeezing the ball between your little finger and thumb, then your ring finger and thumb, middle finger and thumb, and finally index finger and thumb. Do 8-10 squeezes with each finger. These exercises will isolate and develop muscles that need strengthening.

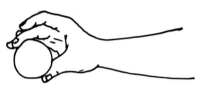

Develop strength and endurance by squeezing the ball many, many times. These squeezing exercises develop neglected muscles that will aid greatly in overall development and prevention of injury. Learn how to develop yourself by *doing*. Be aware of the little things that might help you develop more fully. This is an especially good idea if you use your body to make a living, as does a professional athlete or construction worker. Strengthen your hands and help yourself.

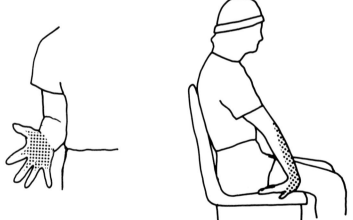

To stretch your hands after squeezing the ball, separate and extend your fingers. Hold for 5 seconds. Do twice. Also, stretch your forearm as shown on pp. 48 and 88. □

BAR DIPS

Bar dips, using your own body weight, are excellent exercises for upper arms and chest. These are tough to do, so don't be discouraged if you can only do a few at the start.

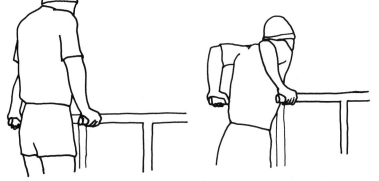

Starting position is with arms straight on the parallel bars. Lower yourself to a 90° bend at the elbows, and return to starting position by straightening your arms. This is one repetition.

Start with what you can easily do for one set, even if you can only do one or two dips at a time. For example, I may be able to do 10 dips once, but after that I would be too tired to do 10 in the next two sets. But if I choose to do 8 in the first set, I will not burn myself out. Then I can do 8 for the second, and 8 again for the third set.

Getting turned off before you get started is usually the result of an approach to exercise that is too drastic. Do not extend yourself to the point where there is a negative effect. This can be a basic cause of *not doing*.

Variation:
Seat Drops

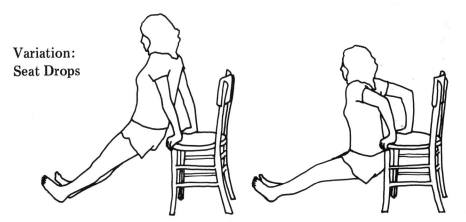

Use a sturdy chair. Start with arms straight, as shown, then bend arms to about 90° or until your butt touches the floor. Then straighten your arms back to the starting position. Start with just a few and gradually work up. These will strengthen the chest and back of upper arms. They are good to do on trips or indoors.

Be careful with this exercise if you have or have had elbow or shoulder problems. □

CHIN-UPS

Chin-ups, or pull-ups, are also a very good natural exercise. They strengthen shoulders, arms, chest and back.

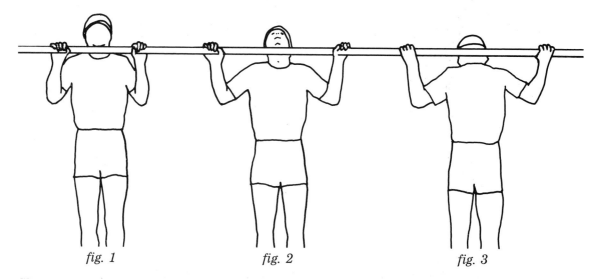

fig. 1　　　　　　　　　　fig. 2　　　　　　　　　　fig. 3

Chin-ups can be done with a forward grip, hands about shoulder-width apart (fig. 1). Or, to develop your shoulders, use a wide grip (fig. 2). A good way to develop the lats (*latissimus dorsi*), the big muscles along the sides of your back, is to do the chins behind your head, using a wide grip. Raise up until you almost touch the back of your neck to the bar (fig. 3.). In all three types of chin-ups, lower yourself to original starting position with arms straight.

Possible Bar Dip and Chin-up Workout: For every three dips try to do at least one chin-up. If this is not the right ratio for you, try two to one, or whatever. The most important thing, again, is to get a workout you can handle, both mentally and physically.

A dip/chin workout could be something like this: three sets of 4 dips and three sets of 2 chins. Alternate the dips and chins—one set of dips, then one set of chins, etc., until you finish. A total of these 18 movements done five times a week would equal 90 dips and chins. Doing these exercises regularly will improve your upper body strength.

The chins and dips are important, but so is your approach in learning how to do things for yourself. Experience is the basis of learning and understanding about yourself and your limits. The enjoyment of staying fit is one of the necessary ingredients of basic human development.

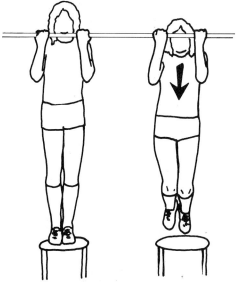

If you are unable to do one chin-up, you can strengthen your upper body by starting the exercise with your chin above the bar. Use a stool to get up to this position. *Slowly* lower yourself. This will greatly strengthen the arm and shoulder muscles. Do several at a time.

Stretches to Use During a Dip and Chin Workout: Do these stretches in between sets. Stretching will allow you to do more repetitions because your muscles will not be as tight.

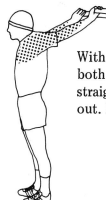

After completing a dip workout, stretch the muscles of the chest and upper arms by allowing your elbows to bend past the 90° angle. Keep your body still as you hang. (Your chest will be about even with your hands.) Hold for 3-8 seconds. A certain amount of strength is needed to do this stretch, so do not try it until you can easily do 12 to 15 dips properly.

With your back to the parallel bars, reach behind you with both hands and grab the inside of the bars. Keep your arms straight behind you. Look straight ahead, with your chest out. Hold 10-20 seconds.

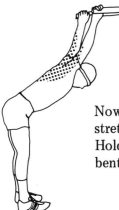

Now face the bars. As you hold the bars with your hands, stretch your back and arms by letting your chest hang down. Hold for 10-15 seconds. Be relaxed. Keep knees slightly bent (1 inch).

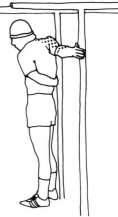

To isolate and stretch the front of one shoulder and arm, face the bars and grab one bar with your right hand about shoulder height. Then, with your left hand, reach behind you and grab the other bar. As you keep your right shoulder close to the bar, look over your left shoulder in the direction of your right hand. By looking over your shoulder, you should get a good stretch in your arm and the front of your shoulder. Stretch both sides. Hold, in a comfortable position, for 10-15 seconds.

These stretches help keep the upper body free of tension and tightness and complement strength development. □

STAIRS

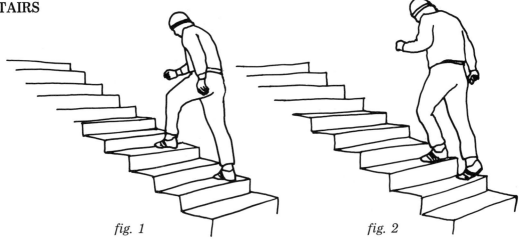

fig. 1   *fig. 2*

Walking and running stadium stairs or steps is a great supplemental workout for the development of strength and endurance. It is a tremendous conditioner of the lower and upper leg muscles, the knees, helps in the prevention of leg injuries, and is a fine cardio-respiratory activity. Even if you run or cycle a lot, you use some leg muscles more fully than others. A workout on stairs exercises many neglected leg muscles. You can find this out for yourself by trying it.

Doing the stairs is a no-pressure workout, a completely individual activity. You do what you can, at your own speed and at your own rhythm. There is no easy way to go up and down. As your legs and heart gradually become stronger, it will get easier.

A stadium is an excellent place for this workout. First you walk the stairs, taking two steps at a time (skip one step in between) to the top of the grandstand (fig. 1). *Walk, do not run.* Use a long stride to pull yourself up. By walking, you increase the muscular strength work by having less forward momentum than you would have by running. Walk at a medium and steady speed to the top; this may be harder than you think. After you reach the top, return to the bottom immediately and start over again.

Come down in a flowing, slightly transversing pattern, not straight down. Coming down straight creates a lot of stress on the knees and ankles.

If you want to *run* the stairs, do so one step at a time without skipping any steps (fig. 2). Make sure you hit each step with the ball of your foot. Then use your toes to push off, driving your knee high, so that you can easily make each step. When running, concentrate on moving your feet quickly. Work on leg speed until you reach the top. Return quickly to the bottom. Be under control. This is a concentrated, continuous-motion workout.

A good supplemental stair workout would last about 30 minutes, but you must gradually work your way up to being able to do this. When you begin a new activity, always start with a workload you can handle. Do not burn yourself out by over-doing at the beginning. Be kind to yourself and gradually develop your strength and stamina, so you are not discouraged by hard work. Before increasing your workload, keep the same stair workout for two weeks, doing it at least three times a week.

I have had a great place to discover the benefits of a supplemental stair workout. While working with the Denver Broncos on rehabilitation, I got into doing the stairs at the Mile High Stadium with several of the players. There it is possible to walk 56 steps or run 112 steps from bottom to top. I usually put in 20 round trips in 30 minutes, which is a fairly condensed workout. (Going up and down the stairs counts as one trip.) Find a stadium or grandstand that allows for walking as well as running steps.

Before and after doing the stairs, stretch your upper and lower legs. You will surely need it.

In your everyday living, walk stairs instead of taking an elevator. It's a vigorous workout for people who want to increase their efficiency in running, walking, cycling, football, track, tennis, basketball, etc. Most athletes benefit greatly by regular activity on the stairs.

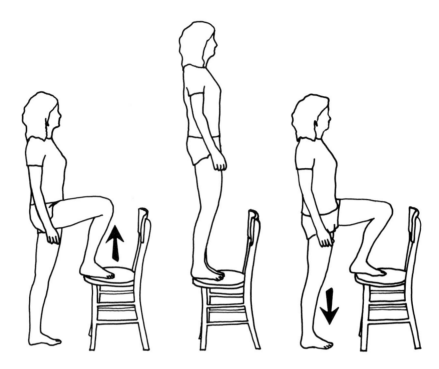

Step ups are also a good workout. Use a sturdy, strong chair or bench, 14-20 inches high. Start at a low height and gradually work up to using something higher as you get stronger. Step with one leg at a time, putting your foot flat on the chair or bench and then bring the other leg up. Almost straighten your legs at the top but keep knees slightly bent (1 inch). Do step ups, starting with right leg first, then left leg. step down one leg at a time. Start slowly and gradually increasing speed as you get used to it. If possible, get to where you can do step ups for 5-10 minutes at a time. Good to do when traveling or when weather is bad. □

Techniques of Running and Cycling

Stretching regularly will open up many opportunities for you. You will be able to run, cycle, ski or swim with greater ease. You will find that cycling helps running, and that running and cycling help skiing, and that stretching will keep you tuned for any of these or other activities. No longer will you have to worry about becoming tight from one activity, and thus cutting down on your enjoyment of another—so long as you stretch and relax.

Running and cycling will develop your endurance and strength and set a foundation of fitness that will allow you to participate in many other activities. On the following pages are some basic techniques.

AT THE BEGINNING

When you start to become physically active again, there are a few things you must realize. First of all, don't work too hard at the beginning. Working hard feels good if you are ready for it. But overdoing it at the beginning can cause mental depression due to aches and pains, and make the thought of more exercise unappealing.

If you do something and do not enjoy it, there is disharmony. A conflict. If you are going to spend time exercising, why not learn to enjoy it as well as improve your physical health? Just be regular with what you are able to do. And as you become more fit and gain more understanding of yourself, you will find that you can work harder and longer than ever before.

Another important aspect of exercise is learning to work within *your* limits. You may think that if you work within your limits there will be little or no improvement. On the contrary, as you learn your present limits, you also learn that it is possible to increase those limits gradually, over a period of time.

With regular positive action, small changes happen every day. The changes may be so slight that you don't really notice them in any one day. It is this accumulation of small, slight changes on a regular basis that leads to natural results. So, if you want to change, do it by being regular with rhythmical activity, stretching, and light, nutritious eating. And without torturing yourself, you will become more energetic, trim, flexible and happy.

RUNNING AND WALKING

If you are just starting to walk or run, do not put a lot of pressure on yourself by thinking, "How stupid do I look?" or "I'm not going fast enough," or "I have to run (so many) miles today," or "I have to run even if I'm tired." Take it easy on your body and mind and do what you feel like doing. Most of us want results now, but getting valuable results takes regularity, without concern about time. We have plenty of time for change, so don't let the thought of time keep you from *doing*. As you become involved with movement, time will pass quickly and soon you will see and feel the changes that come with regular positive action done at your own speed, without pressure.

Before starting a regular routine of exercise, you should have a physical check-up by a qualified medical doctor, which should include a treadmill stress test. This test will help determine your present cardiovascular status during actual exercise. After receiving a doctor's clearance, you can start an exercise program with some self-assurance as to what you can do and what you should do.

Running and walking are basically similar in terms of techniques. The difference is that in walking there is a time when both feet are on the ground at the same time; while in running there is a period of flight (both feet are off the ground at the same time). But still, running is, in essence, an extension of walking.

WALKING

Understanding the basic body movements of walking will help your running. Observe yourself while you walk. Notice the heel-to-toe foot placement. Your toes should point directly forward with each step, with the inner borders of your feet falling approximately along a straight line. Feel how relaxed your upper body is. You have a natural arm swing that starts at the shoulder joint. Your wrists break naturally, and your fingers are slightly curled. On each step, your left arm will move forward as your right leg moves forward and vice versa.

Try walking a distance without moving your arms. This will feel awkward. Now let your arms swing naturally again (directly forward), and feel how this helps your forward movement and balance. Notice that your hands do not come across the midline of your body.

The speed of your arm swing, when walking or running, is directly related to the speed of your legs. Walk faster and see how the speed of your arm swing increases along with your increased pace. Now increase the *length* of your stride and notice how the length of your arm swing increases correspondingly.

When you walk, concentrate on relaxing your hands, arms, and shoulders. Keep an even stride with your head perfectly balanced. Do not take short, then long steps. Just walk at a rhythmical pace, with each step the same as the last. Walk relaxed. Think relaxed. Be relaxed.

TEN WEEK PROGRAM

Here is a ten week program for the person who wants to begin running. It consists of stretching, walking and jogging. (Jogging is slow, rhythmical running.) This will allow you to gradually develop a good foundation of fitness, minimizing the chance of stress or injuries that often happen when you begin running.

The first week, walk one-quarter of a mile a day. The second week, walk one-half mile a day. (Be sure to stretch before and after you walk or run—see pp. 101, 132-33). The third week, increase your walk to three-quarters of a mile, and by the fourth week you will be walking a mile a day. If you walk a mile a day for one year, without increasing calorie intake, you will lose ten pounds; and this ten pounds will stay off because you will have done it gradually, over a period of time.

Walk a mile a day for two more weeks, before you start jogging. An easy way to do this is to start out by stretching, walk one-quarter of a mile, jog one-quarter of a mile, and then walk one-half of a mile. You will still be doing a mile but it will be a walk/jog. The next week stretch, walk one-quarter of a mile, jog one-half of a mile, walk one-quarter of a mile and stretch again. The ninth week, walk one-quarter of a mile, jog three-quarters of a mile and walk one-quarter of a mile. Finally, the tenth week, walk one-quarter of a mile, jog one mile and walk one-quarter of a mile.

A Ten Week Program for Beginners

1st week	stretch 10 min.	walk ¼ mile a day	stretch 5 min.
2nd week	stretch 10 min.	walk ½ mile a day	stretch 5 min.
3rd week	stretch 10 min.	walk ¾ mile a day	stretch 5 min.
4th week	stretch 10 min.	walk 1 mile a day	stretch 5 min.
5th week	stretch 10 min.	walk 1 mile a day	stretch 5 min.
6th week	stretch 10 min.	walk 1 mile a day	stretch 5 min.
7th week	stretch 10 min.	walk ¼ mile, jog ¼ mile, walk ¼ mile a day	stretch 5 min.
8th week	stretch 10 min.	walk ¼ mile, jog ½ mile, walk ¼ mile a day	stretch 5 min.
9th week	stretch 10 min.	walk ¼ mile, jog ¾ mile, walk ¼ mile a day	stretch 5 min.
10th week	stretch 10 min.	walk ¼ mile, jog 1 mile, walk ¼ mile a day	stretch 5 min.

After doing this for ten weeks, you should know how to prepare yourself for physical activity and be able to formulate your own individual workout patterns. You will know the importance of warming up, stretching, rhythms and relaxation, regularity, and exercising by how you feel.

I suggest that you experiment with jogging for another four weeks before you begin running. If you decide to try running, mix it with your jogging and follow the same suggested procedures as the walk/jog program, starting with the seventh week. It may be something like this: jog one-quarter mile, run one-quarter, and jog one-half mile. Do this until you are running a mile with a jog for a warm-up and a jog for a warm-down. There should be at least ten minutes of stretching before and five to ten minutes after each session. You may want to walk for five minutes before you stretch.

After four months of following this program, you will have gradually increased your endurance, lowered your resting heart rate, reduced body fat, become more flexible, developed a good attitude, and enjoyed movement more fully.

HOW TO PREVENT INJURIES

When you start to run, you may suffer from an assortment of aches and pains. You may have problems with your feet, Achilles tendons, shins, calves, hamstrings, knees, or lower back from the constant pounding of running. When a certain part of the body becomes tight or inflexible, then another part will try to compensate for the loss of motion. When this happens, injuries are more likely to occur. Here are some suggestions for prevention of injuries.

1. Build a foundation of fitness. Spend plenty of time walking and jogging before you start a running program. This will accustom your muscles and joints to the stress of straight-ahead movement.
2. Rest when you feel tired. If you run when you are tired, you are asking for trouble.
3. Stretch before *and after* each workout (see pp. 132-33). Running, due to the limited range of motion (as opposed to say, gymnastics or volleyball) promotes inflexibility. Stretching will keep your muscles from getting tight and sore.

SUGGESTIONS FOR RUNNERS' PROBLEMS

1. *Achilles tendons:* Do the stretches on pp. 37, 47, 66, 71, 72 and exercises on pp. 156-59. Stretch only with *a very slight* feeling. It doesn't take much to stretch the Achilles tendons. Wear shoes that keep the heels slightly elevated. Consult a podiatrist if possible, about which shoes are best for you.
2. *Shin splints* (pain in the front of the lower leg): Use the stretches on pp. 46, 74, 159 and the exercises on p. 157. Run on a soft surface such as grass and on pavement as little as possible.
3. *Tight calves and ankles:* Do the stretches on pp. 37, 38, 47, 71, 159.
4. *Tight hamstrings:* Do the stretches on pp. 33-36, 50, 52-56, 74-76, 94, 159.

5. *Lower back or sciatic nerve pain:* Do the stretches on pp. 24-30, 40, 58, 59, 62-67, and abdominal exercises on pp. 152-54.
6. *Feet:* Massage arches and rotate ankles, p. 31. *Note:* Improper foot placement, resulting from faulty foot, knee and hip alignment can be the source of many problems. So if you develop any pain in the foot, knee, hip, etc., that does not go away within a reasonable amount of time, consult a podiatrist with a background in sports medicine.

RUNNING

Running can be an activity for the whole family. It is free. It has no restrictions or limitations. It may be done to help promote a feeling of well-being or to burn off extra calories and stabilize weight. It may help prevent heart attacks and the general feeling of old age. Running helps reduce mental and physical tension and can be enjoyed for a lifetime.

When you start running, your main concern is to do it correctly. By correctly, I don't mean to copy someone else, but to think about and learn the basic techniques for yourself and to let it happen naturally. Speed is not important. But as you become regular with stretching and running, you will be able to run faster and easier than ever before.

Don't force your breathing. Breathe through both mouth and nose. Your head should be balanced between shoulders with your eyes focused a few yards ahead.

Run heel to toe (almost flat footed) with the inner borders of your feet falling along a straight line. This straight-ahead position will help keep knee and foot aligned so your weight can be evenly distributed on the bottom of your foot. (However if you are sprinting, or running up a steep hill, you will naturally be up on the balls of your feet.)

While running, the wrists should break naturally with every swing of the arms. Keep your fingers relaxed and slightly curled; do not make a fist.

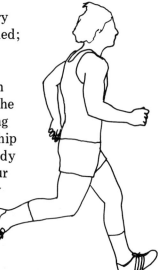

Use your arms to help balance the body so your energy can be directed forward. Bend your arms at a 90° angle, with the lower arms almost parallel to the ground. Your back swing should not bring your hands much beyond the side of the hip bone. In front, your lower arms will move in a slight cross-body direction, but they should not go past the midline of your body. Side movements and body sways only waste energy and make running harder. Be economical with your energy.

Your stride length will depend on your running speed. The faster you run the longer your stride. The slower you run, the shorter your stride. Also, the height of your knee lift will depend on speed. The faster you run the higher your knee lift. And the slower you run the lower your knee lift.

When you are running you may feel the top of your shoulders becoming tight and tense. This means you are losing upper body rhythm. When this happens to me, I relax my shoulders downward and think of weights hanging from my elbows. This keeps my elbows from flaring out and shoulders from tensing, which improves my arm swing. When the shoulders are relaxed, the muscles in the chest are less tense; this allows for easier and freer breathing.

Be aware of how important the arms are for complete body balance and control. The more you concentrate on relaxing your shoulders and arms, the more natural and rhythmical running will be.

To help develop rhythm, stride, and pace in running, practice lifting your knee and pushing off with your toes with each stride. Consciously lift your knee, then use your foot and toes to "grab" the ground beneath you. Then concentrate on "throwing" the ground behind you, using your toes to push off. Be sure to use heel-to-toe foot placement. This will give you added momentum. The emphasis again is on total body balance, relaxation, and rhythm. As you run, think of lifting, grabbing, throwing the ground behind, and pushing off. Do this for several hundred yards at a time. As you concentrate on these techniques you will naturally run faster. Run light and run along a straight line.

Relax as you concentrate on proper, basic techniques. Understand that running is best for you, both mentally and physically, when it feels good, and not when it is painful, or a struggle. When you run, move by how you feel. You will feel different every day—sometimes good and sometimes bad—but if you stretch before running you will find that physical activity is more enjoyable.

Remember to stretch *correctly*. Improper stretching is worse than no stretching at all and leads to injuries. During the past few years I have seen many runners stretch, and most of them do it completely wrong. They bounce up and down or struggle to hold painful positions and call this stretching. What they are actually doing could be called "tearing and tightening." It is only through the controlled, relaxed method of stretching that you will be able to increase flexibility and reduce muscle tension without injuring tissues.

After you stretch, slowly warm up. By warm up, I mean start running at a very slow pace, a jog. Give your muscles time to get warm and your heart time to gradually adjust to the increased workload. Do at least eight to ten minutes of good, slow, rhythmical jogging before increasing your pace. The time it takes to get warm will depend on the temperature outside, and how you feel that particular day. If you start every workout with proper stretching and a gradual warm-up, you will have consistently better workouts and fewer injuries.

On long runs, if you start feeling sluggish and are losing style and rhythm, stop for a few minutes of stretching. Stretch the areas of your body that feel tight. This will help regain the good form, rhythm and energy you need to run efficiently. Many running injuries could be prevented by a short rest/ stretch break taken when needed.

There should be a warm-down period (five minutes of jogging) at the end of each workout. Do not end your workout in a sprint. This is very hard on the heart, which is pumping at a fast rate. It is not very intelligent (if you just think about it) to run hard, then stop. When you run, the blood is needed in the muscles you are using the most—the leg muscles. When you suddenly stop there is a pooling of blood in the legs. So what happens? Without a gradual warm-down period, the blood has difficulty recirculating to the heart and brain because of its weight and concentration in the legs. Ending each workout with a warm-down period will let your heart slowly recover and return to its normal resting rate.

After the warm-down phase, stretch again, when the body is still warm. At this time, stretching is easier. Stretch the muscles that you have just used. Now elevate your feet and legs (see pp. 68–70). Gravity will help circulate the blood back toward the heart and brain. Being in an inverted position will also make the legs feel light again. This, along with stretching will revitalize the body and mind and you will simply "feel good."

Stretching helps you improve and enjoy working out. But the only way to really know this is to try it yourself for at least one month. If you become regular with stretching and exercise, you will improve how you look, how you feel, and what you can do. In that one month you will see that it is possible to reduce soreness and prevent injuries. Your range of motion will increase and working out will become more enjoyable. You will feel better going into a workout and you will feel better when the workout is over. In that month you will find yourself feeling and looking younger.

CYCLING

Cycling is a rhythmical activity that will help keep the upper legs, waist, and hips trim. It is tremendous for the development of the muscles around the knees, exceptional as a strength and endurance builder, and a great off-season conditioner.

Cycling offers a rhythmical activity that helps develop the heart and lungs, without the constant pounding of jogging or running. Because this pounding puts much stress on the body, running rhythm is much harder to develop than cycling rhythm. And for people who just don't like to run, cycling offers a good alternative for health and cardio-respiratory efficiency.

For people already into running, cycling offers a good supplemental workout. As long as stretching is done regularly, cycling will help running and running will help cycling. (See pp. 116–17 for cycling stretches).

To begin with, get a bike that fits you in frame size. To check the frame size, straddle the frame. Your feet should be flat on the ground with the top bar of the frame almost touching your crotch. If the frame is touching your crotch, not allowing your feet to rest flat on the ground, then it is too big for you.

The tilt of your seat should be very slightly upward. Your riding position should be comfortable, with your weight evenly distributed between seat, handlebars and pedals. Your position should allow you to ride comfortably with both arms straight or slightly bent. If your arms are slightly bent at the elbows, you will be able to absorb much of the shock of cycling. This also reduces tightness in the upper body.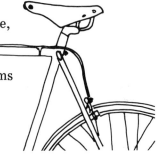

The seat should be high enough to allow for a bend in the knee when your leg is extended. Do not adjust the seat too high, making the leg too straight. Experiment until you find a position that allows for maximum power and comfort. There are many ideas on correct seat height. To find out what works best for you, experiment between a well-bent knee and a slightly-bent knee.

For increased power and stability, use toe clips and straps on your pedals. This will give you the feeling of being a part of the bicycle. The toe clips will keep the feet in a proper, stable, straight-ahead position. This will allow for increased stability and balance with greater distribution of leg power. With toe clips, you have the added dimension of being able to pull up as you ride.

Some Basic Techniques for Cycling:

Getting on and off of your bike correctly is important. Mount by straddling the frame, then put one foot on a pedal and go from there. Do not put one foot on the pedal and then flip your leg over the bike; this causes stress on your bicycle. Likewise, when dismounting, do not flip one leg over as you are coming to a stop. Instead, slowly come to a stop and dismount by removing your feet from the pedals, one at a time, so that you are standing straddling the bike, and then swing one leg over the frame.

When riding, always keep your bike in a straight line, unless you have to avoid something in the road. Your upper body movements should be kept to a minimum; pedal from the waist down. Riding in a straight line will help your balance and forward momentum.

Pedal in a gear that allows for fairly quick leg movement, or approximately 65-85 revolutions per minute. You should feel just a little more than slight tension throughout the entire revolution. To begin with, if you have a ten speed, try riding in either the big gear in the front (chain wheel) and the middle gear in the rear (sprocket), *or* ride in the small gear in the front and the second gear in the rear. (Count the rear sprocket gear with the smallest number of teeth as number one.)

Learn how to operate your gears easily and smoothly and keep your pedals moving as you change gears. Keep the bike balanced in a straight line. Patience is very important when learning to do this.

Help develop rhythm by pulling up on the toe clips and pushing down on the pedals. As you pull up from the toe clips with one leg, push down with the other. This will increase speed and rhythm. Keep this rhythm—pull up, push down. Ride in a gear that allows you to spin the crank and pedals rhythmically.

If you have bicycle shoes and shoe clips (shoe clip attaches the shoe to the pedal), learn to pull back as you pedal. This will help in the development of greater leg strength, and in the feeling of rhythm, as it adds another dimension to technique.

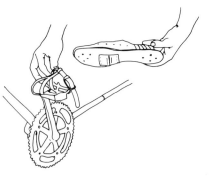

Ankling is an advanced technique of cycling. Start each downward revolution with the heel below the toes. At about the quarter point of the down revolution, use the toes to extend downward (fig. 1), thus providing added momentum and power. As you complete the push-down phase, start the pull-back phase of ankling (fig. 2) and continue to pull back for about a quarter of the up revolution. Sustain the momentum by using your toes (at this point your heels should be above your toes) to pull up on the toe clip (fig. 3). After nearing the top of the pull-up phase, again start the downward phase with the heel below the toes. At about a quarter of the way through the down phase, extend the toes downward, thus bringing your toes below your heel (fig. 1).

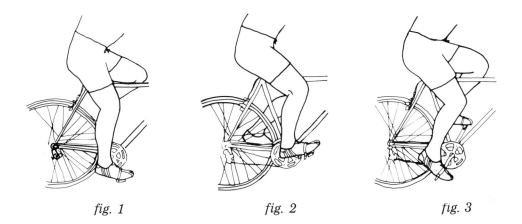

fig. 1   *fig. 2*   *fig. 3*

Learn to push down, pull back, and pull up, as you keep your knees directly over your ankles and close to the frame. Ankling will develop the feeling of "spinning" the pedals and will help in the development of muscular strength and cardio-respiratory efficiency.

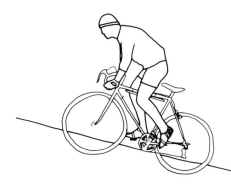

When cycling up hills, you may have to stand up on the pedals for more leg power. As you do this, keep your arms slightly bent. Practice riding this way on flat pavement for a short distance to get used to the balance involved.

You will find it necessary to change to an easier pedalling gear when going up hills. Change gears just before you start to lose rhythm. Always be in a gear that allows for consistent, continuous leg speed without loss of rhythm. Again, keep your knees over your ankles and close to the frame.

Develop a sense of true relaxation as you ride. This will allow you to stay mentally alert. When you are cycling, do not take it for granted that cars, people, or animals will stay out of your way. You must always be on top of the situation and ready for the unexpected. There is no time for daydreaming. For your own survival, be aware of everything around you.

Eight Week Program for Beginners

Cycling can have great benefits. But, as with other types of activity, it may be hard to start and stay with it. The following chart will give you an idea of how to begin.

Since we are all different, the program is open to personal adjustments.

	Mon.	Tues.	Wed.	Thurs.	Fri.	Sat.
1st week	5 min.	5 min.	5 min.	6 min.	6 min.	7 min.
2nd week	7 min.	7 min.	8 min.	8 min.	10 min.	10 min.
3rd week	10 min.	12 min.	12 min.	13 min.	13 min.	15 min.
4th week	15 min.	18 min.	18 min.	21 min.	21 min.	22 min.
5th week	25 min.	25 min.	25 min.	25 min.	28 min.	28 min.
6th week	30 min.	30 min.	33 min.	35 min.	35 min.	37 min.
7th week	40 min.	40 min.	40 min.	43 min.	45 min.	45 min.
8th week	50 min.	50 min.	53 min.	55 min.	57 min.	60 min.

Ride in gears described on p. 176 for the first three weeks. Ride at a pace that allows for rhythm, as you concentrate on your cycling techniques. Do not struggle. At whatever level you start, adjust to slow, gradual increases so that you can develop a good foundation of fitness.

Bike Maintenance for Safety:

Check tires for wear, cuts or small particles of glass which may eventually cause a flat or blowout.

Keep the correct tire pressure. This helps in longer tire wear. Tire pressure will have to be adjusted to the temperature.

Keep your brakes adjusted and replace brake pads when they are worn out.

As much as possible, keep chain, chain wheel, and rear sprocket free of dirt. Do not let these parts rust. Keep the chain oiled, but don't over-oil. Use a kerosene rag and a small wire brush to clean parts. Kerosene will help keep the factory oil on the parts. Do not use a solvent that removes all the factory lubrication. Riding is much easier and smoother when these parts are clean and lubricated.

Always carry a spare tire or inner tube, a pump, water, and a quarter for a phone call with you when you ride. □

Light, Nutritious Eating

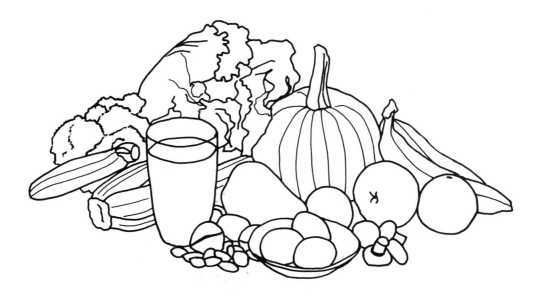

So much has been written about food, with many different ideas and opinions, that it is easy to become confused. One way out of the confusion is to find out what works best for *you*. If you try light, nutritious eating, you will discover that the right amount and kind of food make a difference in how you look and feel.

We should be concerned with how much we eat. Generally speaking, getting heavy simply comes from taking in more calories than are being burned up. The excess is stored as fat. Overeating does not come from true hunger, but is often a nervous habit due to mental tension and boredom. It is a subtle form of punishment disguised as pleasure. But this pleasure is quickly gone once we feel bloated and heavy.

It is good to leave the table feeling satisfied, but not stuffed. While you are eating, try to recognize when you feel satisfied and push away from the table. Don't eat beyond that point. Be aware of your mind and its thoughts. Relax and turn your thoughts to something other than food.

Along with how *much* we eat, we must consider *what* we eat. Today we are conditioned to eating "garbage food" such as potato chips, soft drinks, candy, white bread, adulterated ice cream, goodies from vending machines and fast foods from coast-to-coast chains of hamburger stands. Many of our children have chocolate drink instead of real cow's milk, pop instead of water, and refined sugar desserts instead of fruits. When we are young, our minds become fixed on certain so-called foods, and we develop habits that we will have for a lifetime.

Nutrition and proper eating habits are learned at home, but many parents are not much concerned with the real nutritional value of the food they eat themselves or serve their children. They serve things that are quick to prepare, or they are concerned only with how food looks and tastes.

Sometimes we identify so much with what we eat that if someone says something against our favorite food, we are offended. We are conditioned to eat certain foods and will defend our right to eat them. We feel we won't enjoy life as much if we change our eating habits. This personal identification with certain foods is a barrier to change and experimentation.

You can't change your eating habits in a day, but it is easy to drop one thing at a time. A good way to improve is to stop eating refined, processed, or prepared items. This includes white sugar, white flour, or anything packaged with preservatives (most store-bought crackers, bread, cake and cookies). If possible, avoid fried foods and canned goods (where heat has destroyed much of the food value). Try not to eat snack foods such as soda pop, candy bars or potato chips. If you can do this, your tastes will gradually change. This doesn't mean that you will learn to like things that don't taste good, but rather that as you improve your diet, your taste buds will be able to detect subtle and delicious natural flavors in foods. "Garbage foods" will not taste so good when your sense of taste is sharper. It will no longer be a matter of self-discipline to eat the right foods.

There are lots of recipe books out now on preparing meals with fresh fruits and vegetables, whole grains, nuts and seeds, good dairy products, and lean meat. If you want to be creative you can learn how to substitute whole grain flours for refined white flour, honey, molasses, or date sugar for refined sugar, and fresh produce for preserved, prepackaged and canned goods in recipes you might now use. At first, it may take a little time and practice to prepare healthful meals that taste good and are satisfying, but it's not hard if you have an open mind, do enough research, and use some common sense.

With time, your body will show its appreciation. As you continue to eat the right kind of foods for your individual needs, and exercise regularly, you will feel and look better. Experiment to find out what kind and amount of food agrees with you so you can stay trim and feel light, yet have plenty of energy.

Proper nutrition and regular physical activity can add happiness and youthfulness to your life. Movement is much more enjoyable when your body is getting the proper nutrition daily. Your body/mind will feel energetic when you are not slowed down by heavy foods or overeating. Without a proper understanding of nutrition, you are certain to function far below your personal potential.

Developing Better Eating Habits:

1. Eat only when hungry. Your stomach will call for food when the body needs it.

2. Don't eat between meals. It keeps your digestive system overloaded.

3. Don't overeat. Leave the table feeling satisfied, not stuffed. Chew your food longer. Relax and enjoy your meals.

4. Read the labels of packaged foods you buy. Avoid any with sugar, artificial flavoring or coloring, or with chemicals you can't pronounce.

5. Earn some meals with exercise. Don't just eat for something to do.

6. Miss some meals now and then, especially on days with little or no physical activity. Give your digestive system a rest.

Changing your eating habits is not easy. Have the courage and self-discipline to say *no* to bad habits that destroy energy and health. Learn to live a well-rounded life which combines stretching, relaxation, light eating, work, and physical activity. If you can control yourself, you will develop to your fullest potential, naturally and enthusiastically. □

Caring for Your Back

More than 50% of all Americans will suffer from some sort of back problem some time during their lifetime. Some problems may be congenital, such as sway back or scoliosis (lateral curvature of the spine). Others may be the result of an automobile accident, a fall, or sports injury (in which case the pain may subside, only to reappear years later). But most back problems are simply due to tension and muscular tightness, which come from poor posture, being overweight, inactivity, and lack of abdominal strength.

Stretching and abdominal exercises can help your back if done with common sense. If you have a back problem, consult a reliable physician who will give you tests to see exactly where the problem lies. Ask your physician which of the stretches and exercises shown in this book would be of most help to you.

Anyone with a history of lower back problems should avoid stretches that arch the back, called hyperextensions. This creates too much stress on the lower back, and for this reason I have not included any such stretches in this book.

The best way to take care of your back is to use proper methods of stretching, strengthening, standing, sitting and sleeping. For it is what we do moment to moment, day to day that determines our total health. In the following pages are some suggestions for back care. Also see p. 107.

Some Suggestions for Back Care and Posture:

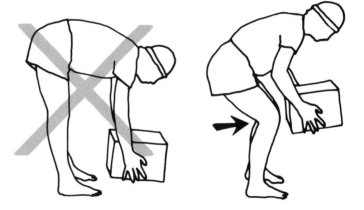

Never lift anything (heavy *or* light) with your legs straight. Always bend your knees when lifting something, so the bulk of the work is done by the big muscles of your legs, not the small muscles of your lower back. Keep the weight close to your body and your back as straight as possible.

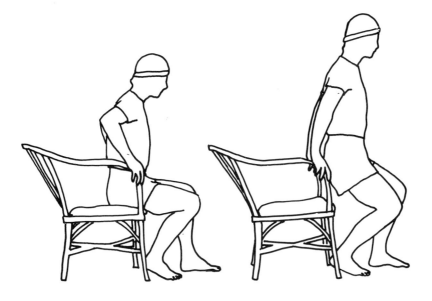

Getting in and out of chairs can be a hazard to your back. Always have one foot in front of the other when rising from a chair. Slide your butt to the edge and, with your back vertical and chin in, use your thigh muscles and arms to push yourself straight up.

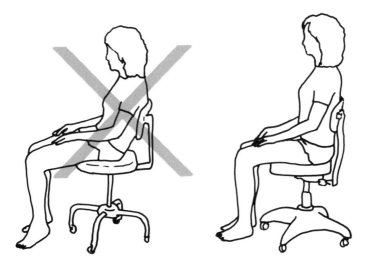

If your shoulders are rounded and your head tends to droop forward, bring yourself into new alignment. This position, when practiced regularly, will lessen back tension and keep the body fresh with energy. Pull your chin in slightly (not down, not up), with the back of your head being pulled straight up. Think of shoulders back and down. Breathe with the idea that you want the middle of your back to expand outward. Tighten your abdominal muscles as you flatten your lower back into the chair. Do while driving or sitting to take pressure off the lower back. Practice this often and you will naturally train your muscles to hold this more alive alignment without conscious effort.

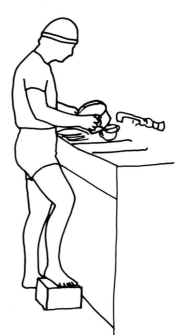

If you stand in one place for a period of time, as when doing the dishes, prop one foot up on a box or short stool. This will relieve some of the back tension that comes from prolonged standing.

When standing, your knees should be slightly bent (½ inch), with feet pointed straight ahead. Keeping the knees slightly bent prevents the hips from rotating forward. Use the big muscles in the front of the upper legs (quadriceps) to control your posture when standing.

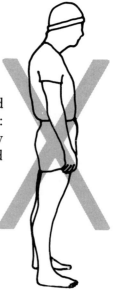

Do not stand with knees locked. This tilts the hips forward and puts the pressure of standing directly on the lower back: a position of weakness. Let the quadriceps support the body in a position of strength. Your body will be more aligned through the hips and lower back with knees slightly bent.

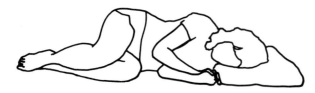

A good, firm sleeping surface helps in back care. If possible, sleep on one side or the other. Sleeping on your stomach can cause tightness in the lower back. If you sleep on your back, putting a pillow under your knees will keep the lower back flat and minimize tension.

When you are aware that your posture is bad, automatically adjust yourself into a more upright, energetic position. Good posture is developed through the constant awareness of how you sit, stand, walk, and sleep.

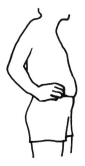

Many tight and so-called bad backs can be caused by excessive weight around the middle. Without the support of strong abdominal muscles, this extra weight will gradually cause a forward pelvic tilt, causing pain and tension in the lower back. Here is a suggested routine to improve this abnormal condition:

1. Develop the abdominal muscles by regularly doing the abdominal workout (ab curl, elbow-knee, and alternating elbow-knee ab curl, pp. 153-54). Again, exercise within your limits. It takes time and regularity. But if you don't get into it, the condition will only worsen.

2. Develop the muscles of the chest and arms by doing the knee push-ups (p. 155). These push-ups isolate the muscles in the upper body without straining the lower back. Start an easy three-set routine like: 10-8-6, or whatever—just get started!

3. Stretch the muscles in the front of each hip as shown on p. 48, and stretch the muscles of the lower back (pp. 24-30 and 62-67). By strengthening the abdominal area and stretching the hip and back areas, you can gradually undo this forward pelvic tilt which is, in so many cases, the main cause of back problems.

4. Slowly let the size of your stomach shrink by not overeating. A person who is overweight needs more food to fill an over-stretched stomach than a highly conditioned athlete who works out regularly.

5. Learn how to walk before you jog, and jog before you run. If you walk a mile a day (at one time) everyday, without increasing your calory intake, you will lose ten pounds in one year. □

Stretching and Exercise Prescriptions

Here is a summary of the stretches and exercises in this book that can be used by health care professionals when prescribing individual fitness and re- habilitation programs. Circle the stretches and exercises that are appropriate for the individual.

STRETCHES

Relaxing stretches for your back · *pages 24-30*

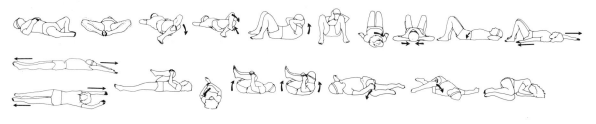

Stretches for legs, feet & ankles · *pages 31-39*

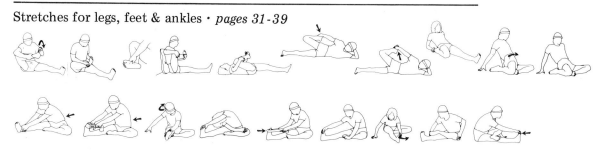

Stretches for the back, shoulders & arms · *pages 40-45*

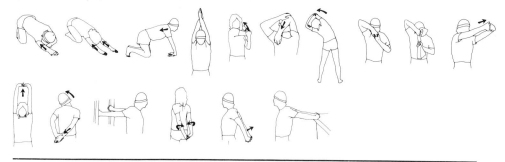

A series of stretches for the legs · *pages 46-51*

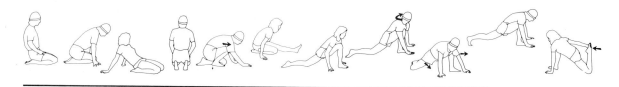

Stretches for the lower back, hips, groin & hamstrings · *pages 52-60*

Stretches for the back · *pages 62-67*

Elevating your feet · *pages 68-70*

Standing stretches for legs & hips · *pages 71-77*

Standing stretches for the upper body · *pages 78-83*

Stretching on a chin bar · *page 84*   Stretches for upper body using a towel · *pages 85-86*

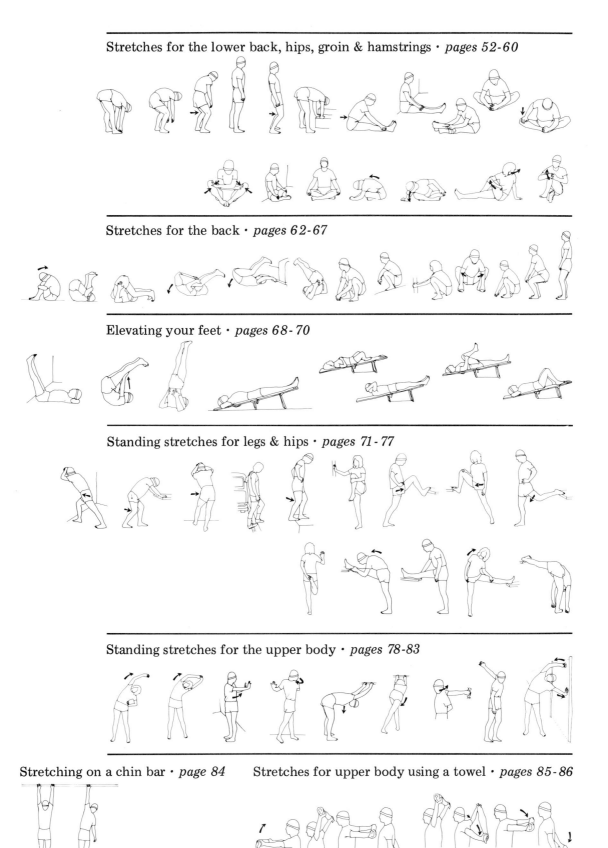

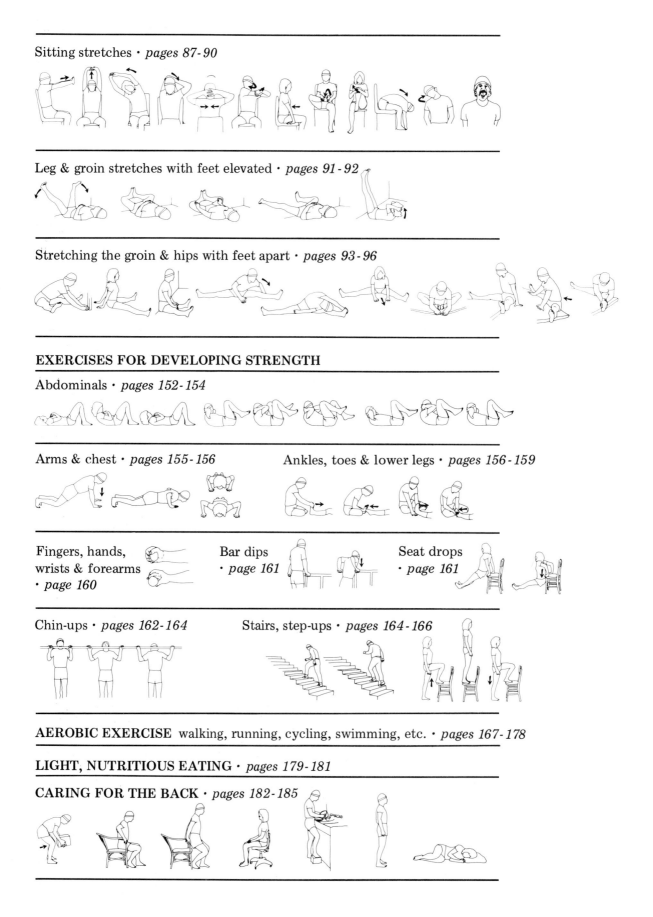

Sitting stretches · *pages 87-90*

Leg & groin stretches with feet elevated · *pages 91-92*

Stretching the groin & hips with feet apart · *pages 93-96*

EXERCISES FOR DEVELOPING STRENGTH

Abdominals · *pages 152-154*

Arms & chest · *pages 155-156*   Ankles, toes & lower legs · *pages 156-159*

Fingers, hands, wrists & forearms · *page 160*   Bar dips · *page 161*   Seat drops · *page 161*

Chin-ups · *pages 162-164*   Stairs, step-ups · *pages 164-166*

AEROBIC EXERCISE walking, running, cycling, swimming, etc. · *pages 167-178*

LIGHT, NUTRITIOUS EATING · *pages 179-181*

CARING FOR THE BACK · *pages 182-185*

Bibliography

Alexander Technique. Wilfred Barlow. Alfred A. Knopf, Inc., New York, N.Y. 1973.
> An interesting technique dealing with harmful habits and the mis-use of the body and its realignment.

Awareness Through Movement. Moshe Feldenkrais. Harper and Row, New York, N.Y. 1977.
> Illustrated easy-to-do health exercises to improve posture, vision, motivation, and self awareness.

Bike Tripping. Tom Cuthbertson. Ten Speed Press, Berkeley, Calif. 1972.
> Highly informative introduction to the proper and efficient use of a bike for transportation and recreation.

Breathing, What You Need To Know. Ruth and Edward Brecher. American Lung Association. 1975.
> Basic facts for the adult reader. A clear grasp of the human breathing system.

The Complete Book of Running. James Fixx. Random House, New York, N.Y. 1978.
> America's best selling running book.

Essential Exercises for the Childbearing Year. Elizabeth Noble. Houghton Mifflin Co., Boston, Mass. 1976.
> A self-help guide in preparing for and recovering from pregnancy. Straightforward instructions, good illustrations.

Foot and Ankle Pain. Rene Cailliet, M.D. F. A. Davis Company, Philadelphia, Penn. 1968.
> A clear, concise guide for diagnosis and treatment of foot problems written for doctors and physical therapists.

Guidelines to Successful Jogging. Rory Donaldson. National Jogging Association, Washington, D.C. 1977.
> A practical approach for joggers.

Healthful Eating Without Confusion. Paul Bragg, N.D., Ph.D. Health Science, Santa Ana, Calif. 1975.
> A short book on various diets. Clearly and simply written.

Helping Yourself with Foot Reflexology. Mildred Carter. Parker Publishing Company, Inc., West Nyack, N.Y. 1969.
> Of general interest. Shows how to manipulate the reflex "buttons" located in the feet.

Hypokinetic Disease, Diseases Produced by Lack of Exercise. Hans Kraus, M.D. and Wilhelm Raab, M.D. Charles C. Thomas, Publisher, Springfield, Ill. 1961.
> This book deals with problems caused by lack of activity. Fairly technical.

The Knee in Sports. Karl K. Klein. Jenkins Publishing Co. The Pemberton Press, Austin and New York. 1976.
> Helpful information on conditioning, injury prevention, rehabilitation, and studies related to the knee.

Knee Pain and Disability. Rene Cailliet, M.D. F. A. Davis Co., Philadelphia, Penn. 1973.
> Written for doctors and therapists. Illustrated; stress is on functional anatomy.

The Knees: Growth-development and Activity Influences. Karl K. Klein. Jenkins Publishing Company, The Pemberton Press, Austin and New York. 1976.
> A very good book on growth and development and the influence of activity on the knees.

Low Back Pain Syndrome. Rene Cailliet, M.D. F.A. Davis Co., Philadelphia, Penn. 1969.
> A practical text for medical students and physical educators.

The Massage Book. George Downing. Co-Published Random House, New York, N.Y./ The Bookworks, Berkeley, Calif. 1972.
> Clear, concise methods of partner and self-massage.

Mucusless Diet Healing System. Prof. Arnold Ehret. Ehret Literature Publishing Co., Beaumont, Calif. 1972.
> About eating foods that do not cause mucus. Late 19th-century style writing.

New Aerobics. Kenneth Cooper, M.D. Bantam Books, Inc. New York, N.Y. 1970.
> A basic book on the importance and application of daily aerobic exercise.

Oh My Aching Back. Leon Root & Thomas Kiernan. New American Library, New York, N.Y. 1975.
> A guide to back pain and various things you can do about it.

Prevention and Treatment of Running Injuries. John Pagliano, D.P.M. To be published 1980.
> A noted running podiatrist discusses and recommends ways to deal with problems of running.

Richard's Bicycle Book. Richard Ballantine. Ballantine Books, Westminster, Md. 1972.
> Bicycle selection, riding, touring, racing, elementary maintenance, history, lore, and general enjoyment. Presented clearly in an inexpensive volume.

Run, Run, Run. Fred Wilt. Track and Field News, Inc., Los Altos, Calif. 1965.
> A good book by several authors (and one of the earliest) about the mechanics and training methods of running.

Runner's Medical Guide. Richard Magni, M.D. Simon and Schuster, New York, N.Y. 1979.
> One of the best books available on runner's problems.

Running Free. Joan Ullyot, M.D. G. P. Putnam & Sons, New York, N.Y. 1980.
> Expands and compliments the social changes produced by running. Excellent for women.

The Shocking Truth About Water. Paul Bragg, N.D., Ph.D. Health Science, Desert Hot Springs, Calif. 1975.
> Impressive facts and simple explanations about the necessity of pure water for good health.

Super Brain Breathing. Paul C. Bragg, N.D., Ph.D., Health Science, Santa Barbara, Calif. 1979.
> Excellent book on breathing exercises and the importance of oxygen. I do these exercises every day.

Touch for Health. John F. Thie, D.C. DeVorss and Co., Santa Monica, Calif. 1973.
> A practical guide to natural health using acupuncture, touch, and massage.

Treatment of Injuries to Athletes. Don H. O'Donoghue, M.D. W.B. Saunders Company, Philadelphia, Penn. 1976.
> Over 800 pages of illustrations and detailed text. A textbook for doctors, physical therapists and physical educators.

Track Technique. Fred Wilt, Ed. Track and Field News, Inc., Los Altos, Calif.
> A good resource for physical educators. (A quarterly publication).

Van Aaken Method. Ernst van Aaken, M.D. World Publications, Mountain View, Calif. 1976.
> One of the world's leading experts on endurance training and health discusses fasting, women and running.

About the Authors

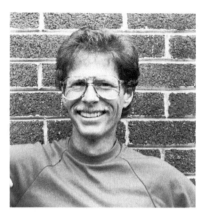

Bob Anderson was born in 1945 in Fullerton, California and is a graduate of California State University at Long Beach, with a lifetime teaching credential in physical education. He has taught stretching to the Denver Broncos, the New York Jets, the California Angels, the Los Angeles Dodgers and the Los Angeles Lakers; set up stretching programs for the football teams at Southern Methodist University, University of California at Berkeley, Washington State University and the University of Nebraska; has taught emotionally and physically handicapped children; worked with executives at the North American Rockwell Space Division; taught professional rodeo riders, as well as swimmers, cyclists, weight lifters, tennis, racquetball, handball, and volleyball players. He has also worked with members of the U.S. Olympic Ski and Figure Skating teams, and for the last seven years has taught stretching at the Pikes Peak High Altitude Running Camp in Colorado.

In 1968, at the age of 23, Bob began a personal physical fitness program, since he felt he was overweight and out of shape. He changed his diet, started eating less, and began running and cycling. His weight went from 190 to 135 pounds over a period of time, and he soon was in much better physical condition. One day, while in a conditioning class in college, he discovered he could not reach much past his knees in a straight-legged sitting position. After discovering how tight he was, Bob started stretching. In several months he became much more limber; he found that stretching made running, cycling and other activities easier and more enjoyable and that it eliminated most of the muscular soreness that usually accompanies strenuous physical exertion.

After several years of exercising and stretching with Jean and a small group of friends, Bob gradually developed a method of stretching that could be taught to anyone. Soon, he was teaching his technique to others. He began working with professional teams, then college teams, other amateur athletes, and with a variety of people at sports medicine clinics, racquetball clubs, athletic clubs and running stores throughout the country.

Bob and Jean first published their book *Stretching* in 1975 and in four years sold over 35,000 copies by mail. Articles on their stretching techniques have appeared in *The Runner, Runner's World, Powder:The Skier's Magazine, Swim-Swim, Down River, Esquire, Playboy, Organic Gardening, House and Garden, Glamour,* and *Vogue.* Bob's public appearances created such a demand for information on stretching (8,000 letters received after his first appearance on *The Today Show)* that in 1979-80 this revised version of the book was published. Bob has recently toured Japan and Germany, conducting stretching workshops. *Stretching* has been translated into eight foreign languages.

Jean Anderson was born in 1945 in Long Beach, California and has a B.A. in art from California State University at Long Beach. She began running and cycling with Bob in 1970. She developed a system of drawing the various stretch positions as she and Bob worked on the different stretches through the years. Jean was the typesetter, illustrator and editor of the first edition of *Stretching.* She also designs, hand-dyes and knits multi-colored wool hats. Bob and Jean live with their daughter Tiffany in Palmer Lake, Colorado. □

Index

continued . . .

... Index

Credits

Editor
  Lloyd Kahn, Jr.
Consulting Editor
  Charlotte Mayerson
Art Director
  Drake Jordan
Typesetting
  Sara Schrom
Pasteup
  Helen Jordan
  Susan Sanders
Proofreading
  Susan Friedland
  Marjorie Jacobs
Printing
  Mo Shallat
  Sunset-Recorder Press
  San Francisco, Calif.
Photostats
  Joseph Fay, Marinstat
  Mill Valley, Calif.
Headlines
  Headliners
  San Francisco, Calif.
Typesetting
  IBM Electronic
  Selectric Composer
Typeface
  Century
Book paper
  60 lb. Lowell Wove Offset

Acknowledgements

Thanks to the following who, in one way or another, helped make this book possible:

Carlton Anderson • George Anderson • Kathryn Anderson • Tom Anderson • Art Berglund • Arnold Bryman • Bill Buhler • Roger Cannon • Herman Clayborn • *Co-Evolution Quarterly* • Paul Comish • Lesley Creed • Tom Dunn • Tom Ferguson • Steve Garvey • Tom Gienapp • Vince Gomez • Steve Hartt • Allen Hurst • Greg & Cathy Johnson • Dr. Karl Klein • Mark Lomas • Rudy Meoli • Dr. John Pagliano • Dr. Bill Patterson • Jim Pursell • John Ralston • Don Rowe • Nolan Ryan • Bill Shepard • Rod Sherman • Ed Shipstad • Mike Simone • Bill & Ginny Singer • Annette Smith • Dr. Ed Souter • Larry & Joyce Staab • Otto & Judy Stowe • Del Tanner • Lou & Jeanne Tramantano • Dr. Art Ulene • Bill Wright

More On Stretching

From Bob and Jean Anderson

STRETCHING CHARTS

22½ x 34" wall chart

Stretches to do before and after:

Aerobic Exercise	Racquetball/Hand-
Badminton	ball/Squash
Baseball	Rodeo
Basketball	Running
Curling	Skiing (Downhill)
Cycling	Soccer
Everyday (General)	Softball
Figure Skating	Swimming
Football	Tennis
Golf	Triathlon
Gymnastics	Volleyball
Ice Hockey	Walking
Martial Arts	Wrestling
Motocross	X-Country Skiing

17 x 22" wall chart

Specific stretches for:

Boardsailing
Bowling
Computer & Desk
Groin/Hip
Kids
Legs
Lower Back
Neck/Shoulder/Arms
Over 50
Partners
Pregnancy
Rowing
Surfing

Excellent visual aids for group or personal use

$3.00 each (folded, packaged) + shipping: $1.00 per chart, 20 cents ea. add'l. chart

Special laminated charts — durable, attractive — write for prices.

STRETCHING CHART PADS

To fill the needs of the medical profession, coaches or anyone wishing to distribute charts as a handout to groups at clinics, races or workshops, our charts are now available in a reduced size at a lower cost.

8½ x 11" pads of 40 identical sheets, printed both sides

$6.00/pad + shipping: $1.00 per pad, 20 cents ea. add'l pad.

STRETCHING CARDS

Set of 16 pocket-size cards (4 x 4½")

Currently available for:
Running, Everyday, Travellers and Cycling
(More to be published soon. Send for catalog.)

Easy to carry with you anywhere.

$3.95 ea. set of 16 cards + shipping: $1.00 per set, 20 cents ea. add'l. set

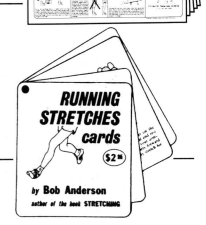

STRETCHING WORKSHOPS

If you are interested in Bob Anderson lecturing or conducting a stretching workshop for your group or organization, write to the address below.

To order, or to write for a free catalog, send to:

Stretching Inc., Box 767, Palmer Lake, Colorado 80133

More Fitness Books From Shelter Publications

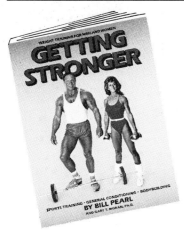
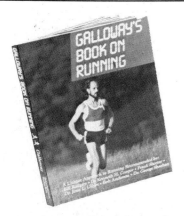
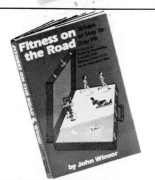